RUNNING THE ENDLESS RACE

finding *something runderful* in
a world with no finish line

Ally Robinson

Running the Endless Race:
finding something runderful in a world with no finish line

© 2024 Ally Robinson

This book was *not* written by Ally's mom. *iykyk*

ISBN 978-1-961185-64-7 (paperback)
ISBN 978-1-961185-65-4 (hardcover)
ISBN 978-1-961185-66-1 (ebook)

Cover Photo courtesy Jeffrey Vanags – ***www.jeffvanags.com***
Modeling Photo on page 32 courtesy **Valvic Photography**

Cover Design, Editing & Layout: Megs Thompson – *in omnia paratus publishing llc*

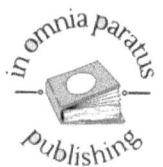

www.inomniaparatuspublishing.com

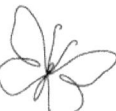

This book is dedicated to every little girl who's ever felt like they were unworthy, to the women rediscovering themselves after embracing their role as a mother, and to the runners who continue to push through, not only their marathons and daily training, but this endless race we call life.

For so long, I was afraid to tell my story. The thought of turning my experiences into a full-length book for the world to read was even more daunting. But here we are, and this book exists because of the unwavering support and belief of so many incredible people.

Thank you to my dear Megs, who guided me through the overwhelming publishing process and brought this book to life. Your expertise and encouragement made all of this possible.

To Dawn, my best friend, thank you for standing by me through every step of this journey. Writing a book is no easy feat, but your constant reassurance made this process more bearable and less lonely.

To David, thank you for reminding me that sometimes 'no,' means not yet. Thank you for not taking no for an answer, and coming back time and time again until I told my story.

To my husband Donny, who held me so tightly that all my broken pieces could heal, thank you. Your love mended what was shattered and gave me the strength to keep going.

And to all the friends and family members who walked with me through the darkness and stayed long enough for me to find the light, this book is as much yours as it is mine.

Thank you for believing in me when I struggled to believe in myself.

TABLE OF CONTENTS

 # Introduction

I never thought I would be sharing my story. Honestly, my story still might have been locked deep inside my soul forever if it hadn't been for a man named David Covington. David had been coming to me for years asking if I would tell my story for a film he was putting together about suicide awareness.

But in my mind, attempting to kill yourself was something shameful and should be hidden. Or, as I was told after my attempt, *that I am a middle-class white girl and have nothing to be depressed about.*

But David knew me as a girl. My dad worked for him; we would go to his house for company parties. My dad was a hard-working guy; he never missed a day of work. So, it was strange when, on a Monday morning, he left David a voicemail to inform him he would not be coming in that day. David called him back, joking and teasing about why he was calling out for maybe the first time ever. My dad just responded. *"Well, actually, David, Ally attempted to take her own life, and we still aren't sure if she is going to make it."*

My dad worked in the mental health field. He had been leading a suicide prevention workgroup for the last two years; how could this be happening to his daughter? But that's the thing: it can happen to anyone. Yes, even a 15-year-old girl.

Even though I desperately tried to move past that portion of my life, David still followed me through social media. He watched me grow up, as I proudly shared pictures of my husband and son on Facebook. He watched as I found my passion and purpose in life, creating my own successful online business as a running coach.

David reached out to me about a documentary-style film he was putting together. He asked if I would be willing to share my story for the film. I told him no, absolutely not. A year later, he reached out again. I finally agreed to a phone call, strictly out of respect for my dad's boss.

David passionately told me about the other speakers he had lined up for the film and how they were people from all walks of life, like the marine who found himself on a dark path after a tragic plane accident. Still, they didn't have a tenacious young woman who could be the voice for teenagers struggling with mental health. I countered with, *"David, I do not want to tell a story about a depressed teenage girl who took a handful of pills."* He responded, *"No, Ally. This isn't the story of a depressed teenager who tried to commit suicide. This is a story about how you found life. You get to tell this story however you want."* No matter how well David painted the picture of his passion project, I still politely declined to participate in his film.

But his words kept circulating in my mind: *a story about life.*

The fear of judgment and shame has continued to stop me from sharing my story and the lessons that I have learned from coming out of my darkest moments. I'm a running coach. My entire career is based around the fact that I'm a support system and cheerleader for my clients. My job is to inspire, motivate, and help them to achieve their big goals. How in the world would they still trust and look up to me if they knew the truth about my past or my struggles with mental health?

But then I found myself suffering in a race… Mile 30 of a 33-mile Ultra Spartan. An obstacle course race with not only a lot of miles to run but also a lot of obstacles, 60 in total. And through the suffering, cramping calves, bleeding hands, and utter exhaustion, I just kept thinking about all of the hard things I had already gone through in life. Right there in the middle of the race, I cried in pain and gratitude that I was still alive to do these hard things. If my clients want to achieve their goals, they must know that their past, their story, and their hardest moments will help them push through to the next level.

And so, over a year later, David once again messaged me. *"Holy smoke, you won your age group in an Ultra Spartan?"* I knew that something in me was changing, something big. The entire story that I'd been telling myself for as long as I could remember, the things that I was ashamed of, the things that made me angry, sad, and frustrated. The things that made me feel unworthy. Those experiences and emotions were actually my strengths, and my clients needed to hear that. And so, when he mentioned for at least the third time, *"Ally, this would be an amazing story to integrate into the Moving America's Soul on Suicide Film,"* I replied, *"David, I have a story to tell."*

David and I arranged for him to fly to Miami to capture my story. At the last minute, something came up, and he couldn't come. Instead, the very first time I ever told my story, a story that not even my husband knew the entirety of, I was in a hotel room with not one but two complete strangers… with two video recorders capturing my every word, to be produced and turned into a film for the entire world to see. After two full hours of spilling my guts and baring my soul to these strangers (who now knew me better than anyone else), I remember walking out of the hotel and sitting in my Jeep. A huge wave of relief washed over me, the tightness in my chest finally relaxed — like I had just left pounds of trauma, hurt, and sadness behind in that hotel room. Thanks to that film, *Moving America's Soul on Suicide*, I finally had the courage to write this book.

In the following pages and chapters, I will tell you my story: I will detail the events that led to my suicide attempt. I don't believe in trigger warnings. Horrible things happen every day. While I will touch on some dark matters, I want you to remember that this book is not just about depression and a suicide attempt. This book is about life. Life, running, and making the choice to keep moving forward.

Amid my darkest moments, it was easy to believe that my story had reached its conclusion—that the pain and despair I felt were insurmountable obstacles that left me with no will to continue on. But running and Spartan racing taught me otherwise. Obstacles were meant to be overcome; if you fail, you do your penalty and keep going.

I started running to keep a goal on my horizon. I could not succumb to the darkness inside of me until I crossed the finish line of a marathon. I woke up early every morning to train. In fact, for the first time in my life, I looked forward to waking up. When I finished my first marathon and they put that medal around my neck, I knew my entire life had just changed.

In the world of running, the finish line is a tangible milestone, a moment to celebrate after miles of sweat, tears, and determination. But the concept of a finish line is far more elusive in life. There is no definitive endpoint, no ultimate destination where we can declare victory. Instead, life is an endless race, a journey of continuous growth, discovery, and evolution. In racing, the goal is always the same, to get from point A to point B as quickly as possible. However, we don't come into this world just to die as quickly as possible. The beauty of the endless race, of actually living life, is to slow down, enjoy the little moments, experience everything you can, fall in love, snuggle your babies, and to savor that first sip of coffee in the morning.

We don't find our purpose in life; we create it. Each step we take, all the choices we make, and every obstacle we overcome are opportunities to shape our destiny. And though the road may be long, I take solace in knowing that with each new day comes the promise of new beginnings, new possibilities, and new reasons to keep running the race of life.

Welcome to… The Endless Race… Where There Is No Finish Line.

Ally Robinson

Growing Like Mold

I am going to start by saying something absolutely bonkers: I was born without the will to live. I know that sounds dramatic. And I wasn't technically suicidal as a little girl. But when other kids talk about growing up, they talk about going to college, getting married, becoming a doctor, lawyer, or the president of the United States. If you asked me what I wanted to be, I'd just lie and tell you I wanted to be a photographer. My mom had a professional camera, so that seemed to be an appropriate answer. For as long as I can remember, I've had this little voice in my head that told me I would never see the day when any of that grown-up stuff would happen for me. It's like I had blinders on. I couldn't see anything further than what was right in front of me. Which is problematic when that means you don't care about the consequences of your actions or have any regard for your future.

When it came to homework, for instance: I NEVER did my homework. Man, I would get into so much trouble with my teachers. Why bother with homework? Why do something I didn't want to do if I was never going to graduate high school or go to college? Why study for tests if my grades didn't actually matter?

But I wasn't just some delinquent. I was a really good kid growing up with mousy brown hair and freckles. I was always the shortest girl in the class… with probably the biggest personality. I've always loved performing on stage, whether that was dancing, singing, or starring in plays. I loved the spotlight! At a young age, I started performing in *The Nutcracker*, which quickly blossomed into a love affair with ballet. And if you know anything about ballet, it's a serious commitment, especially for a young girl. Ballet practice 5-6 nights a week in addition to any dress rehearsals or performances, it was easy to say that ballet took up most of my free time and became a big part of my identity.

I grew up in Phoenix, Arizona. At that time, my parents were still seemingly happily married. I was the oldest of four kids, two brothers, and a sister. Our household even included a dog and a couple of cats.

My dad was a senior director of adult services in the mental health field. I didn't know what that actually meant when I was a kid, so in my child-like mind, I understood this to mean that my dad managed the people that managed the people that helped the *"crazy"* people. *Please don't cancel me over my insensitive and childlike view of mentally ill adults. Again, this was what I thought when I was little, based on the conversations I overheard between my parents. Like most kids, when I heard about facilities for mentally ill people, I thought about the things you saw in movies: people in straight jackets and padded rooms, mumbling incoherently and trying to eat bars of soap.* The only thing I knew for sure was that my dad worked really hard to help people. And out of all the jobs he could work really, really hard at, he chose to help the mentally ill and maybe even *"crazy"* people who needed help. So, I admired my dad. Though he worked long hours, he still made time to sit and color with me (even though he was color-blind). We would go swimming together on the weekends. Dad would jump off the diving board while simultaneously tossing me in the air so I could have those few seconds of feeling like I was flying before plunging back into the water with a splash. He would read me bedtime stories, like *Stuart Little*, while I cuddled my favorite faded pink blanket. My dad would even take me horseback riding in the Arizona Desert.

My mom left her position as a therapist and crisis worker (where she initially met my dad) to start a small home daycare. There, she could wrap her entire life around us kids. She always put her kids first, ensuring we had fun activities to fill out our days.

Mom was always planning something fun to keep us kids busy and entertained. I remember days when she would help us make a fort so we could have a camping adventure in the living room or pull out all of our craft supplies to spend the afternoon creating something new.

Because my mom had a home daycare, I got to wake up every morning and spend the day with my friends. The party was always at my house, and I became the natural ringleader. For better or worse, as long as my mom had her daycare, I had a steady stream of best friends all the time. I never worried about fitting in or whether or not people liked me. Even when I would put on my prettiest princess dress and strut around the house, no one judged, they just joined the fun.

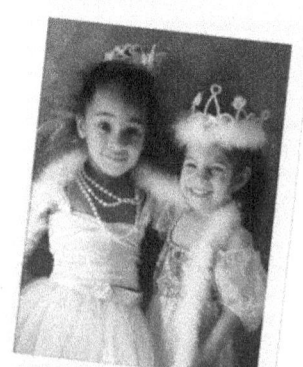

I remember one morning, super early, Mom woke me up and quietly escorted me to the car. I did as I was told and promptly fell back asleep. When I woke up again, we were in California and headed for Disneyland. There's nothing quite as magical as waking up in the parking lot of the happiest place on earth.

All dressed up with my best friend.

By all accounts, my childhood was perfect.

When I was in 3rd grade, we moved to the epitome of white picket fence suburbia. It was a large middle-class house with 5 bedrooms, an upstairs, and a finished basement. It was the middle of the school year and the girls my age already had their friend groups established. While they weren't outwardly mean to me, I could tell that I wasn't exactly welcome. What can I say, girls talk, and hearing that you're considered different or uncool can hurt. The fact that on my first day at my new school, I chose to show up in an ankle-length bright pink sequin skirt, bell-sleeved white lace top, and clicky little heels while everyone around me was sporting tee shirts, jeans, and Converse probably didn't help. I started believing the narrative that girls are mean, no one likes me, and I was never going to fit in. This narrative followed me for the rest of my childhood, and I often struggled to create meaningful connections with other girls my age. I felt like I was always on the outside looking in and could never seem to break this cycle.

But I didn't need friends, my mom was my best friend. We spent hours lying in bed watching movies and reruns of *Little House on the Prairie*. Although she no longer had her home daycare, my mom did get a really fancy camera and occasionally did photoshoots for newly engaged couples or families. I always came along as her assistant, holding the reflector and blinding the models when I shined the light right into their eyes.

I wasn't just helping mom with her photoshoots, though. Early in her pregnancy with my youngest brother, mom had to be put on bed rest due to super-premature contractions. At the time, I was 10, my brother was 6, and my sister was 2. As you can imagine, having such young children at home made it difficult to follow all of the doctor's orders when it came to being on full bedrest. Yet, I did what I could to help. It was around this time that my dad started filling his free time at home with work and becoming less involved with the household, so I also stepped in as an emotional support for Mom. I rubbed her neck and feet and was a shoulder to cry on when things were rough. A year later, when mom dislocated her shoulder (for the second time) and had to have surgery, I once again took over helping out as much as I could around the house.

As close as my mom and I were, she never really knew how I was truly feeling, how lonely and cast out I felt in my friend group. I always wanted to be there for her, to help in any way I could. But I knew that talking about my feelings or emotions would be burdensome, so I just hid them away. After all, Mom was pretty busy with 4 young kids running around the house.

That house my family bought, the one with the 5 bedrooms and a basement. Well, it came with a secret. A secret lurking under the new flooring that was just installed before we moved in. The first time it rained, boy, oh boy were we in for a surprise. The valley of Phoenix is known for being incredibly hot and dry, rarely ever raining. Welcome to the desert. On the rare occasion that it does rain, it's like the heavens open up and pour buckets upon buckets of rain that can last hours or even days during monsoon season.

On one of those rainy nights, the basement flooded. Water seeped in through the walls of the basement, creating a mini swimming pool in the lowest level of our house. My mom and I stayed up late in the night trying to shop-vac the floors, dump out the water, and continue the process again and again and again to avoid the new hardwood floors from getting ruined. While all of this was going on, my dad was upstairs sleeping, completely unbothered by the flooding basement. So, Mom and I were busy tackling the issue alone. My parents had people come out to figure out where the leak was coming from, and they tried a couple of things to fix it. But every time there was a heavy rain, water came flooding in. This happened again and again, every time it rained, over the years we lived in this house. My mom and I spent countless nights shop-vacing rainwater out of the basement, stopping only when my baby brother woke up and needed to be rocked back to sleep. It was exhausting, and really hard work, but my mom needed me, so I helped.

My little sister, Zoe, was born a fighter. And by fighter, I mean she was born purple and not breathing. Which is fitting for someone we have affectionately called "*Wheezy*" most of her life. My sister, from the beginning, had an array of health issues. But being wheezy in a house prone to flooding was a danger none of us could have imagined.

Mold grew up on the insides of the walls of our house. Aspergillus is a common mold that can cause health issues. And we lived completely unaware of the toxic danger lurking and wreaking havoc on the health of the whole family. Weird things started happening, like when I lost my sense of smell for a few years. Mom could have pulled a batch of freshly baked cookies out of the oven, and I couldn't smell a thing. Our cat, Heidi, lost her ability to meow; she'd open her mouth to cry, but nothing came out. My mom developed terrible asthma and seemingly constant allergic reactions. But the person that got it the worst was Zoe.

One of the scariest parts about Aspergillus is that under the right conditions, in the right person with a weakened immune system, Aspergillus can grow in the lungs, causing serious health issues. Unfortunately, this is exactly what happened to my little sister. At such a young age, she became a victim of this mold, carrying it around in her lungs like a walking greenhouse, which set off an autoimmune response in her little body, adding to her already scary health issues.

It took countless different tests and hospital visits to diagnose the issue and then extended hospital stays to administer steroids in hopes of helping Zoe fight this battle. Sometimes my mom and sister would be gone for days, if not weeks, in the hospital.

When I was in middle school, my sister had one of those extended stays in the hospital. My grandmother (my dad's mom) came to stay with us so she could help with the kids and watch my youngest brother, Logan, who was about two at the time, while my other brother and I went to school. One morning, as I was getting ready for school, my grandmother told me that she had to leave. She didn't tell me why or when she would get back. She just walked out of the house. I stood there confused, wondering what I should do. My dad had already left for work, and my mom and sister were at the hospital. I walked my brother to the bus, figuring that at least one of us should get to school on time, and I stayed home to watch Logan. I called my best friend Matt's house and talked to his dad. When I explained what was happening, he offered to drop Matt off to spend the day with me, to keep me company, and to help me watch my baby brother.

This was the day of our school dance. All day while playing silly toddler games with my brother, I was excited to get all dressed up and go to the dance. When my dad got home from work, he dropped me and Matt off in front of the school. Once we got inside, though, we found out we weren't allowed to join the fun in the gymnasium because we'd missed school that day. This is just one of the many childhood experiences I missed out on because I was trying to help take care of my family.

My grandmother never came back. In fact, that was the last time any of us saw her. Like, ever. After a petty argument with my parents during an incredibly stressful time, my grandmother found herself so incredibly offended that she decided to walk out of our lives forever. In doing so, she left me and my brothers to fend for ourselves until Dad got home from work that evening. I don't think I'll ever understand how she could do that to her son and her grandkids. I guess she didn't care about us.

Because I was forced to be incredibly mature for my age, I stepped up to the plate to help raise my brothers. I was responsible for and did get my younger siblings ready for school, packed lunches for all of us, made dinner, and tucked my siblings into bed. No one asked me to do these things or thanked me for it; I just did what wasn't being done by the adults in our lives.

I was resentful of my sister; it was all her fault that our life wasn't as picture perfect anymore. I was mad at my parents because they weren't around as much as I wanted or needed them to be. When my mom was home, she was consumed by caring for my sister with around-the-clock breathing treatments.

As much as I resented Zoe, as a big sister, it was my job to protect her. It didn't seem fair. My sister was so sick, on breathing treatments and steroids, in and out of the hospital, just a little spitfire of messy curly hair fighting for her life. And here I was, healthy, and couldn't care less about my own life. She stole my mom away from me. She took all the attention with her medical needs; she stole my childhood while I was stuck taking care of my brothers… And yet. If I could have laid down my life and given her my healthy body, I would have, in a heartbeat.

Instead, I started to self-destruct.

I felt unappreciated and desperate for the love and attention all children need from their parents. I missed the relationship I'd had with my dad before. I longed for the days when we spent time together, when he prioritized me and he would do fun things with me, like take me to the midnight premiere of one of the Harry Potter movies. Instead, when he was home, he was either locked away in his office or watching sporting events on TV. Worse was when my mom was gone running errands. Then he yelled about how messy the house was. He rage cleaned, slamming kitchen cupboards, and stomping on the floor while my siblings and I hid upstairs, hoping he would forget that we existed.

What none of us realized at this point was that the mold found in our basement had grown inside the walls of our home, all the way up to the top of the second floor. As a family we hadn't noticed any big changes, because we had become nose-blind, but when we would leave for a weekend and come home, we started noticing an odor when we opened the front door. We also started seeing weird black spots growing on the vaulted ceilings of our entryway. We learned that those black spots were connected to the mold that had started in the basement, climbing its way up inside of the walls. The only way my little sister was going to get better or even survive, was for us to get out of the house as quickly as possible.

Because of how much mold had grown in the house, there was no way it could be sold. My parents had no choice but to foreclose on the house. It was a mad rush to pack up everything, find a new house, and move. Just like when we were dealing with the flooding of the basement, all the work of moving fell on me and Mom. The two of us strained our muscles moving mattresses, dressers, and even my dad's heavy wooden desk. In the end, anything we weren't able to get out in time was locked away in the house and lost forever.

Titanic

As kids, we were led to believe that my dad was just busy at work. He was always away, or busy, and it seemed like his job consumed all his time. Now, as a parent myself, I realize the harsh truth: he wasn't just occupied with work. He didn't want to face the stress of our move, the foreclosure, or the heaviness of having a sick and dying daughter. He chose to distance himself from the overwhelming weight of our family's struggles.

At 12 years old, I didn't know much about love and relationships, but I knew one thing for sure—I didn't want a marriage like my parents had. My dad was the provider, the one bringing in the money, but there had to be more to a partnership than just financial support. I saw my mom, day in and day out, exhausted, stressed, and often at her wit's end. She bore the brunt of everything, from managing the household to taking care of us kids, all while dealing with her own deep feelings.

I tried to be there for her, to offer whatever emotional support I could, but I was just a child. I couldn't fill the void that a loving husband should have filled. I remember lying in bed with my mom, talking late into the night, while my dad was downstairs watching TV. She seemed so sad, so lonely, so worn out. Despite being many years younger, I could relate to her feelings.

It's not that I didn't love my dad. I loved him very much, but I felt so protective of my mom. I didn't want her to hurt anymore.

I remember begging my mom to get a divorce. I told her that together, we could figure out how to make ends meet and raise the kids without my dad. I believed we could find a way to survive, just the two of us. We were a team. But she wasn't ready to make that transition. She wasn't ready to let go of the life we had, even if it was filled with heartaches.

Eventually, the relationship lines between Matt and me blurred and he became my boyfriend. *If you can even call someone a 'boyfriend' at such a young age.* We shared a love for books and music. His dad would pick us up and take us to this really cool arcade that had go-kart racing and laser tag. His family went out of their way to really make sure that I felt welcome, even inviting me to attend his niece's baptism. It was a breath of fresh air to see a father so involved with his kid's lives. He understood the medical issues my little sister was going through, and he was compassionate about the stress I was under. Matt's dad really took me under his wing and was almost a second father figure to me. He bought me Starbucks gift cards and brought me ice cream at school. Those little tokens of affection made me feel loved and special. While my own dad reminded me to brush my hair a hundred times a day (because he apparently thought the only way I'd be successful is if I looked pretty enough to snag a rich husband), Matt's Dad constantly reminded me that I was intelligent and talented. That I had value in just being me.

I was heading into my troublesome teenage years, and as Matt and I were about to start high school, we started to grow apart. His dad got upset that we no longer hung out. He would constantly text me to try to talk me into dating his son. As irritating as that was, he was also one of the only adults in my life that I felt like I could talk to.

Because my mom was often gone dealing with Zoe's medical issues, and my dad was always working, I had a lot of freedom to get into things that I otherwise wouldn't have been able to. I felt unappreciated, misunderstood, and lonely in life. I found solace in the attention of teenage boys, sexting, and promiscuous behavior. I lost my virginity on my 15th birthday, way before I was ready to handle the emotional implications of sex. And the guilt and shame that came with that ran deep in my veins. I couldn't look at myself in the mirror. I hated myself.

I knew if the family that I loved so much knew the things I was doing, they would be heartbroken… but I couldn't stop. I could, however, talk to Matt's dad about these things, and it never felt like he was judging me. He never lectured me, and always made sure I was safe, whether that meant taking me to get condoms or even buying me a pregnancy test once when I was too scared to do it myself. My cell phone stopped working right before I was supposed to go to summer camp one year, and Matt's dad immediately picked me up and took me to the store to buy me a new one.

I came to realize that this wasn't an innocent father figure and daughter relationship, no matter how much I wanted it to be. He started to tell me things like *"I love you,"* in a way that was anything but fatherly. He also began to tell me how jealous he was of the boys I was dating, how much better he would be at taking care of me, at loving me. He would send me graphic sexual text messages. As much as I wanted to tell him to stop, to tell my parents, or go to the police, I knew I couldn't. He knew all of my dirty secrets. I feared that if this one aspect of my hidden life came to light, then all the other things I was hiding from my parents would surface.

Thankfully Matt's dad never touched me, at least not outside of forcibly holding my hand as he drove me home one day. At the height of the *#metoo* moment, I was thankful that my own situation had never gotten that far. I was never in a situation where I was intoxicated beyond being able to consent. I never screamed *"no"* only to be ignored. Most of my sexually promiscuous behavior involved me throwing myself at one boy or another, in hopes of gaining love and attention. But even then, it wasn't always welcome attention. When news got out that I was *"easy,"* it just opened the door for more teenagers to coerce me into doing things I wasn't comfortable with. I found myself in a nightmare situation when I sent a partially nude photo of myself to someone that I trusted. That picture then started circulating amongst my classmates, completely shattering any self-respect I had left.

I started dressing differently. Long gone were the days of pink sequined skirts and clicky little heels. I would have given anything for a do-over. I wore baggy pajama pants to school, black jackets, and oversized hoodies even in the peak of Arizona's heat. I hoped that these clothes could hide my small frame, swallow me completely, and hide me away from my shame. This behavior, and these experiences, ate me up inside. The self-hatred I felt ran deep, and I didn't know how to stop the pain I was feeling.

I tried self-medicating. I hoped that by taking a variety of different pills, I would find something that would numb the pain. Most of everything just made it worse. And the pills I could purchase with the little bit of cash I got a hold of weren't always what I thought I was buying. A couple of times, I ended up getting really sick from the medication I blindly consumed. One time the pills I took made the floors move so badly that when I tried to walk, I puked up this vile orangish-yellow substance. That orangish yellow toxic waste stained my hands and feet for weeks, where it had touched my skin. I can only imagine what it had done to my insides.

I started to fantasize more and more about death and dying, all while dancing ballet for several hours after school every day and trying to balance the trouble I was getting into and maintaining the perfect helpful daughter image I was still desperately trying to hold on to. Everything about my life was going downhill fast. It felt like I was trapped in the last hour of the movie *Titanic*, where confusion and desperation took over. People were running around, screaming, while the ship continued to sink.

I thought it was best that I kept all of this turmoil inside. Though I was internally screaming, I didn't want anyone to hear. I knew that I needed help. I was a danger to myself. I felt like I needed to be locked up. I knew deep down that I needed to be taken away to one of the facilities my dad worked with. I needed to be put into a straight jacket and placed in a padded room. I know my parents started seeing the signs, but I was the master of manipulation and learned at an early age that being a chameleon kept everyone around me happy. So that's what I did. I made excuses. I lied. But, at the end of the day, I still couldn't see any light at the end of the tunnel for me.

Around this time is when I knew that I was going to end my life. I didn't know how; I didn't know when. But I knew I could not live with who I was. It was like everything I had ever felt as a child was finally making sense. I was never supposed to grow up. I would go down with the ship.

3, 2, 1 KaBoom

Like a quietly ticking time bomb, a 15-year-old girl can only be so sneaky before all the lies and deceit come to light and, metaphorically, explode. It didn't happen overnight. There were calls home to my parents, talks with the school counselor, my grades plummeted, and my mom even cornered me, demanding I take a drug test. The *good girl* facade I was putting on was cracking and falling apart fast. I was desperate to keep up appearances. I never wanted my parents to know that their darling daughter was doing the things I had been doing behind their backs. Then, the local authorities got involved. They had to reveal to my parents that they had discovered an explicit photo of me online. My cell phone was taken away, I was grounded, and I felt like my entire life was over. That was when the real Ally, the one I'd been hiding, was uncovered, and the illusion of the wonderful, obedient, and helpful daughter they'd thought they had, was lost forever.

The breaking point for me was when my mom sat me down to have a serious conversation. She wanted to know what was going on with me. We'd been so close, and I was her best friend. She told me everything. What she didn't realize was that our relationship only went one way. I wasn't telling her anything about what I'd been thinking or feeling for a very long time. There was so much she didn't know about who I was. It was at that moment that I realized I didn't think I could handle the consequences of my actions. The embarrassment, my ruined reputation, the shame, the added stress I'd caused my family. Those bad decisions would certainly follow me for the rest of my life, and I didn't want to have to live with those ramifications.

I wasn't afraid of dying. I needed a do-over. And, being raised Buddhist with a belief in reincarnation, I believed that dying meant a fresh start. Of course, it also meant that I would come back to a life without my siblings, who I loved so much. They were the only reason I hadn't tried to kill myself sooner. But now that my family hated me, sticking around was only going to do more harm than good.

Friday, I knew it was going to be my last day of school. I only showed up to spend time with my friends and my favorite teachers, to say goodbye in the only way I thought I could without giving away my plan. I skipped all of my least favorite classes because it seemed stupid to spend part of my last days on Earth sitting through lectures in subjects I was already failing. After the school day was over, I went to ballet rehearsals as usual. It was midway through class when my mom stormed in and dragged me out of the studio. She'd received a call from the school, letting her know that I'd skipped classes throughout the day. My mom was not just broken-hearted but angry at this point. She was ready to pull me out of school completely. She realized that something big needed to change if there was any hope of me straightening out and getting my act together. But what she didn't know was that I'd already decided something big was going to happen. I had no intention of ever going back to school.

On Saturday morning, my dad woke me up and told me to get dressed. We were going to the grocery store. Without them saying anything, I knew their plan was to keep an eye on me at all times. They were going to keep me from getting into any more trouble than I already had. We picked up supplies to make brunch for the family: French toast. As we stood in line at the checkout counter, I remember thinking that it sounded perfect for one of my final meals. I looked longingly at the selection of candy. I am not much of a chocolate person, but if this was going to be my last day on earth, I thought I might really miss York Peppermint patties. *"Dad, can I get a Peppermint patty?"* *"Of course, kid,"* he responded.

I ate that chocolate-coated mint patty slowly, trying to memorize how my mouth felt cool and tingly when I breathed in. I knew this would be one of the last sweet treats I ever had. The realization forced me to turn my head and wipe away a stray tear as I finished every bit of my peppermint patty on the drive home.

At the house, I gave my siblings all the love and attention I could. They probably caught more red flags than my parents that day because even though I loved my siblings more than anything, I certainly didn't go out of my way to spend time with them outside of my usual big sisterly duties.

It's so silly to note this next part… but I really want you to understand the workings of my 15-year-old mind. Before dinner, I did my makeup and hair, trying to tame my frizzy, now red-dyed hair. I guess I figured that when my parents found me dead the next morning, it would be slightly less shocking if I looked pretty. I wanted to look like I was just in a deep, forever sleep. Like *Sleeping Beauty* in the movies. While we were eating, my mom commented aloud, comparing me to a porcelain doll.

When it was time to say goodnight to my family, a part of me wanted to hug them each a little longer, but I didn't want to raise suspicion. I went to my bedroom, turned off the light, and got in bed, pretending to fall asleep. I lay there thinking about what I needed to do. It was like I was going through a to-do list in my mind. Checking off the things I knew needed to be done before I took my last breath. I tried to keep any thoughts of fear or hesitation out of my mind. *Would it hurt? Who would find my body?* Anytime these thoughts popped into my head, I tried to remember that my parents, my entire family, were going to be better off without me there. I would no longer be messing things up and ruining their lives. My mom already had enough stress on her plate with my younger siblings, my sister's health concerns, and the fact that my dad was pulling further and further away from the family. She definitely didn't need the headaches and heartbreaks that I was bringing into her life.

Once the house was quiet and everyone else was asleep, I got out of bed and started writing letters. I wrote them to people who honestly wouldn't have cared about receiving a dead girl's final words. But even after I died, I wanted someone to care about me because I couldn't care enough about myself.

I put all of the letters in a yellow box and placed it next to my bed.

I walked softly into the kitchen, to the family medicine cabinet, and grabbed what I thought would be a lethal dose of prescription drugs. Just to be sure, I made a quick Google search on the family computer and confirmed that the pills I'd collected would do the trick. Of course, Google also advised that using alcohol to wash them down would be better, but my parents didn't drink, so the pills would have to be enough. I didn't even bother to delete my search history. I'd be gone before they found it anyway.

I held all of the differently shaped and colored pills in my hand, and before I could think about what I was doing, I put the entire handful of pills in my mouth. Immediately I gagged, afraid I was going to vomit before I could even swallow them, I spit the pills out onto the counter and took them again, one by one by one… With each pill I swallowed, I became more sure, more confident, that what I was doing was good. That this was the right decision for me, for my life, for my family.

I knew the drugs would start taking effect before long. At least, that had been my experience in the past with taking large quantities of pills, so I walked quickly back to my bedroom. I laid down on my bed, closed my eyes, and went to sleep, perfectly content that I would never wake up again.

3, 2, 1 Kaboom.

Ally Robinson

 # The Dream

I've never had stage fright before. Singing, acting, or dancing—each performance was a chance to shine, and I thrived under the spotlight. My ballet teacher often praised me for my stage presence. "You sparkle," she would say, pointing out the little flourishes in my movements, the radiant smile that lit up my face, and the expressive gestures that added flair to my performances.

Yet, here I was, on a grand stage, under a glaring spotlight that turned the audience into a sea of darkness. The familiar rush of adrenaline that usually accompanied my performances had turned into a disorienting sensation.

It was like a bomb had gone off, shocking my brain and my senses, leaving my ears ringing and me struggling to find my bearings. I was overwhelmed, confused, and clear-headed all at once.

I stood there, waiting for the music to cue my dance. I strained to hear the familiar notes that would guide me through the routine. The Nutcracker? Perhaps a variation from Sleeping Beauty? But there was nothing.

I stood there in the spotlight, frozen with fear and confusion. I could just imagine the audience staring at me with puzzlement, worry, maybe even amused by my uncertainty.

Panic seized me as minutes stretched into eternity under that blinding spotlight. Fear and confusion mingled, paralyzing me in place.

In that moment, the only instinct that remained was survival. Without a second thought, I bolted from the spotlight, fleeing towards the comforting shadows of stage left. The darkness of the wings enveloped me like a protective cloak.

And everything faded away...

I still don't know if what I went through was what people call a *near-death experience*, a vivid dream, or a crazy mishmash of my brain's attempt to make sense of what I'd just done by using things I recognized from my life. Something so familiar, like my love for dance and performing. I doubt I'll ever know for sure.

 # Walking Among Coyotes

I expected hell to be fiery, with demons. Instead, it was utter darkness. I couldn't move, speak, or even open my eyes. Voices I recognized echoed around me, but I couldn't place names to them. I could hear the voices talk about me like I wasn't even there. *But I'm right here. don't they know that?* I could feel the nurses quickly and aggressively jostling me around as they gave me a sponge bath. I wanted to tell them to stop, but I was stuck inside of myself.

Later, my mom shared with me that while I had been unresponsive in the hospital, anytime she was by my side, the machines I was hooked up to showed a steady calm heartbeat. However, when she got up to leave, even just to grab lunch after spending hours in the hospital room, things would start beeping, registering that my heartbeat had increased. Like, somehow, a part of me knew she was there. That no matter what I had done in the past, I still loved her, and needed her there with me. A silent plea, *please don't go.*

During my hospital stay, there was so much uncertainty. Initially, they were worried I might not make it, but then they started to worry that even if I did survive, what would my cognitive ability be? Would I suffer any long-term consequences?

My first signs of life happened when a voice I recognized stood by the bed, and I felt her caress my hand. With all my might and determination, I squeezed back…

Four days after I swallowed the combination of pills, I finally awoke. I had suffered a cardiac arrest. According to the doctors, I was lucky to have pulled through; If I hadn't been a healthy 15-year-old, I probably wouldn't have survived. Didn't they understand that I didn't want to be here?

The morning of Sunday, March 27th, 2011, my parents found me in my bed. I was unresponsive, foaming at the mouth, and I had urinated on myself. *So much for trying to look beautiful and peaceful in death.* In a panic, my dad picked me up, carried me to the car, and rushed me to the ER.

While I was in the hospital, with Mom by my bedside, Dad went home. I guess fatherly instinct had told him to check the computer search history. That's when he discovered that my overdose hadn't been a reckless accident but instead an intentional suicide attempt. He went to my bedroom looking for anything else I might have left behind and was met with my box of letters.

Shortly after I woke up, the hospital wanted me transferred to a behavioral health unit. I could hardly sit up in bed, let alone walk, because of some neurological issues that resulted from my suicide attempt-induced cardiac arrest. Yet the hospital insisted that I was fine to be transferred. My dad, still working in the mental health field, was familiar with the different recovery options available. He was already worried about this move, but the facility had assured my parents they were ready to take care of me and assist in my recovery. I was loaded into an ambulance bound for a mental health facility. Unfortunately, their inability to properly care for a teenager who was unable to walk at all became apparent only after I arrived.

They put me and my parents in a small room to officially admit me to the facility. Intake was a blur, with the staff asking at least a hundred questions, all while I was dealing with a throbbing headache that made it impossible to focus. I was so exhausted all I wanted was to go to bed. When I was fully admitted, I had to say goodbye to my parents.

Because I couldn't walk and the facility was not equipped to deal with someone in my condition, the best they could bring me was a walker. Two people in scrubs stood on either side of me as I gripped the handles of the walker and attempted to hold up my own weight. I was still wearing my hospital gown, and my blue grippy socks brushed the floor as I shuffled my way across the room.

Every step was excruciating. My arms shook, and I struggled to remain upright as my feet slid against the carpet. Just a few days before, I was dancing in the ballet rendition of *Sleeping Beauty*. Now I could barely hobble across the room.

I just wanted to lay down and die.

That's when anger set in.

Why am I still here? Why didn't I die? Why did I have to fail? Again.

The questions buzzed in my head. *What if I had just taken a few more pills? What if I got a hold of alcohol to wash down the pills… would that have been enough to end my life?*

The scrubbed strangers continued to lead me down this long, never-ending green hallway as tears streamed down my face. I couldn't keep going. I needed to sit down; I needed a break. I was so weak and so tired, but they kept ushering me forward down the long, endless green hallway.

Walking down that hallway was the hardest thing I have ever done in my entire life. It felt like a punishment for failing to kill myself. Just as agonizing was the realization that I was going to have to keep living… And this hallway was the first of many challenges I had to face.

After passing through several locked doors that required key cards to enter and exit, we reached the end of that green hallway. They showed me to my room and helped me into bed. My stay at this mental health facility in the Coyote unit had officially begun.

I woke up early the next morning. I'm unsure what time it was because we weren't allowed clocks in our rooms. We weren't allowed anything in our rooms besides a bed, nightstand, and bathroom with a partially clear shower curtain.

I had to pee, but when I looked around my room, I realized my walker was nowhere in sight. I tried to get out of bed to walk to the bathroom, but I could barely lift myself into a sitting position, let alone trust my legs to carry me.

So, I laid in bed crying, wishing someone would help me to the bathroom to relieve my bladder as time slowly ticked by.

Eventually, a blond woman with long, bright red fingernails came in and helped me to the bathroom. She also gave me a cup and told me I needed to be drug tested. She stood in the room and turned around to give me some semblance of privacy as I produced a sample.

She was nice enough to help me get dressed out of my hospital gown and into the clothes that had been left for me. The pajamas that I wore the night I tried to kill myself. There'd been no time for my parents to go home and collect other clothes, so the hospital had washed my pajamas and sent them with me to the facility. I was grateful to have clothes to wear other than the hospital gown but being forced to continue to exist while wearing the same green pajama pants and white form-fitted t-shirt that I had just tried to take my life in seemed like a cruel joke. At this unit, we weren't allowed to wear shoes, I guess because shoelaces are deadly. So, they gave me a pair of hospital-sent socks: gray crew socks with rainbows on them. *What an oddly chipper sock selection for someone who feels utterly hopeless.*

The lady was kind enough to help me walk around the room to help me regain my strength. I still needed the support of a wall to keep me upright, so I asked for my walker. My request was declined, and I was told that I needed to walk independently to regain my strength.

When it was time for breakfast, I held onto the wall as I was escorted down the green hallway towards food. As I made this maiden voyage, I got my first glimpse of the other teenagers held hostage with me in the *looney bin*. I had just as many questions about them as I am sure they had about the redheaded girl clinging to the wall for life.

Because it was my first 24-hours, I wasn't allowed to eat breakfast with the other kids. They brought me to an isolated room with a tray of food. The breakfast was probably some variation of eggs, a sausage link, and Jello. Because that's what we ate nearly every morning during my stay.

23

A different lady now sat across from me, urging me to eat. My head still throbbed, and my stomach was all in knots. I was starving, but physically I could not bring myself to actually eat. I struggled to get down some of the Jello and sat quietly, waiting to be told what was next.

I guess my not eating raised some red flags because I was labeled with some form of eating disorder. For the rest of my stay, the employees at the *nut house* took extra interest in anything I ate, which was annoying when all I wanted to eat was Jello. You try waking up from a drug-induced coma and being forced into a modern-day asylum and see if you are excited to scarf down food.

After breakfast, the rest of the teenagers and I were brought into the main common area of our unit and put into circle time. We were told to share our names, ages, and why we were there. I quickly learned that while my fellow coyotes had dealt with suicidal thoughts, self-harm, drug addictions, and schizophrenia, I was the only patient who had actually made a serious attempt to take my own life. The fact that I had nearly been successful was apparent when they saw me struggling to stand up or walk on my own. As we all know, kids can be cruel, and the Coyote unit was no different. I was approached by one girl who aggressively demanded to know why I was so pitiful, so weak, and why I looked so sad. When it was my turn to share with the group, I told them honestly about what I'd done, and that I'd just woken up in the hospital before being brought here. My voice got stuck in my throat, and tears welled up in my eyes as I spoke. It's one thing to know what happened, it's another to verbalize it to a group of your peers.

After circle time, that same girl came back up to me. *"Wow, you have some serious balls you actually tried to take your life, and by the looks of it. You came pretty close."* Another kid told her to piss off on my behalf, which I was grateful for, but he then quietly agreed, *"You do have some balls."*

As an attention-seeking teenage girl, it seemed like a huge compliment, a little recognition for my fearlessness. To have been the only Coyote who did the damn thing. But I realize now that playing a game of who got closer to death is not the title I want to be *"king"* of, especially when we are talking about male anatomy.

That evening, when the other teenagers got called to visitation, my heart sank when my name didn't get called. *I guess my parents really didn't care. I really should have tried harder to kill myself. No one cares anyway.* Only later did I realize that you aren't allowed visitors in that first 24-hour period. This would have been good information to have at that time.

My parents did come to see me for visitation the next evening. While they were overly excited to see me, I was petrified of actually seeing them. I wanted them to want to see me, but I didn't necessarily want to see them. I was scared of how they were going to react, what they were going to say, and how much trouble I was going to be in for what I had done. In a desperate attempt to ease the tension, I told them how the other teenagers responded to my suicide attempt. *"They said I have serious balls for actually going through with it."* My parents were less than amused.

Life in a *psych ward* is not so bad. There is Jello, karaoke, team-building games, more Jello, and basketball. I even made a few friends. Maybe I wasn't the only broken teen misfit. My time in the Coyote Unit really helped me feel less alone in my struggles with mental health.

In a couple of days, I was back to my normal self and could fully participate in all the activities. Twice a day, we would go to an indoor basketball court. There we were supposed to move around and, I guess, exercise. Being a 5-foot girl, the shortest in my class, basketball was never a sport I picked up on. But here in the *madhouse*, I had nothing better to do with my two thirty-minute time chunks than learn.

My first attempts at shooting hoops failed. One of my new friends laughed as he effortlessly nailed every ball he threw. He tried to teach me… but it was just one of those things where I had to make my own mistakes over and over until it clicked. After a couple of days, I tossed basketballs like a pro and even won a game of Around the World before my time was up with the Coyotes.

Once I had recovered physically, as much as I had a new love for basketball and Jello, I certainly didn't feel like staying trapped in a *mental health facility* forever. So, I inquired about how I could get my parents to check me out and take me home. I found out that there was a man that came to the unit periodically and would meet with the adolescents and sign off on whether or not they are rehabilitated enough to leave. I found out that I was scheduled to meet with the *"Big Man"* later that day. So, I came up with a strategy in my head. It was, I thought, the perfect plan.

I went into his office quite confident and said, *"Look, if I'm not going to die, then I should probably start living. Being stuck here definitely isn't living. My mom needs me. My siblings need me. And I'm not doing any good for anyone in here."* I was super shocked when he simply sat there, jotted some notes, and casually informed me that he would see me a couple of days later… What the heck?

Later that day, we were allowed to go outside to this fenced-in patio area for some fresh air. I was talking to another Coyote about what a jerk the *Big Man* was. He disclosed to me that he was actually going home later that day. HOW???? How the heck was he going home? I was way more mentally sound than he was. There was absolutely no way he should be going home before me. But then, he gave me the secret.

"You have to tell the Big Man about how excited you are about your future. Tell him about your goals, dreams, ambitions, and all the things you look forward to. That's what I did, and he immediately signed off that I could go home."

As he left the unit, I watched my friend walk down what I now know they call the *Green Mile* as a free man.

I started to form a plan. I had only had a couple of days before my next meeting with the *Big Man* to show him that I was all better. I had to show everyone here that I had a life and future I looked forward to. I requested a pencil and paper to use in my room, and after much persuasion, they finally agreed. I guess they figured they knew me well enough to know I probably wasn't going to try to kill myself by jamming a dull pencil into my eye.

Back in my room, I started writing a poem...

I've walked among Coyotes, but now it's time to be reborn and take into the world all the things I've learned...

I shared the poem with the adults in charge of the *teenage psych ward*, and they absolutely loved it. They even displayed it in the common area for everyone to read.

After a couple more days of art therapy, basketball, and Jello, I was finally ready to meet with the *Big Man* again.

I told him how excited I was to dance in *Sleeping Beauty*, how I looked forward to being a professional ballerina and potentially going to Chicago for a Summer Intensive Program. I explained how grateful I was, that after everything I had been through, I was still healthy enough to dance and follow my dreams.

The *Big Man* seemed happy with that response, and I was sent home the following day. 10 days after being admitted into the behavioral health facility, I was finally a FREE person again.

But I still wasn't actually FREE.

I went from one jail to another... Home became house arrest. I was taken out of public school. No phone, no friends. I was allowed to go to dance practice and come straight home.

Surviving is Not the Same as Living

I went back to being the perfect daughter. I appeared to be helpful and happy. When I returned to ballet rehearsal, of course, everyone was wondering where the heck I had been for the last two weeks. When I disclosed my suicide attempt to one of my friends, a girl on the level above me overheard my whispers, hearing bits and pieces of my story. She piped in with a disgustingly snotty tone," You *are a middle-class white girl. What do you have to be so depressed about? Obviously, it was for attention."*

I never told anyone about my attempt after that. I mean, she was right. My life was good. I had nothing to be depressed about. The fact that I had been, and still was unhappy was embarrassing.

Shortly after I got home from the behavioral health unit, the night terrors started. Every time I closed my eyes to sleep, I had weird, twisted nightmares. It was always the same two dreams, both equally terrifying. In the first nightmare, I had been restrained in a windowless, dark room with nothing but the flickering light of a single wax candle and desperate screams. For what felt like hours, maybe even days, I heard those screams, and they were coming from my loved ones: my mom, my baby sister. . . and the more I struggled to get free to find and help them, the louder and more anguished the screams became. All I could do was watch the wax slowly drip down the side of the candle and listen to the tormented cries of those I'd spent my life trying to help.

In the other recurring dream, I was walking down the long green hallway. As I walked, old friends, ex-lovers, and even enemies lined the walls. When I tried to speak to them, they never acknowledged me. I didn't exist to them, even though they were right in front of me. I was left wondering about the green hallways. Every turn or open door resulted in yet another green hallway. Eventually, I would wake myself up from crying in frustration.

It was weird because these dreams terrified me, but they also made me feel alive. Every morning, I woke up relieved that the dreams were gone. But by evening, I looked forward to going to bed to relive the nightmares. That should have been a sign that I was still mentally struggling, but I wanted to believe that I was better or at least getting better. I didn't know it yet, but that darkness I had inside of me would always be there. Maybe I should have spoken to my therapist more about all of this.

Because of my attempt, I was required to go to therapy with a woman named Vivian. I expected her to be clinical, in a dress suit, with white-gray hair pulled up into a neat bun, and glasses perched at the end of her nose that she'd look through when writing notes about me. But that didn't describe Vivian at all. Vivian was young with a friendly smile, not some impassive old woman. She had short, chopped brown hair, and wore casual clothes. She looked like someone who could be your neighbor or a friend you'd meet for coffee. Far more approachable than the *Big Man* at the behavioral health unit.

On my first day of therapy, she had me sit down on the couch across from her.

Hi Ally. Do you know why you're here?

No. I'm fine. Life is fine.

Well, then, can you tell me why your parents would like us to speak?

I guess, I mean, I took a handful of pills and had to spend a few days in a looney bin…

That's definitely something we could talk about.

Yeah, but like I said, I'm fine. Life is fine. I didn't die, so I'm just trying to get back to living life.

Okay, so, if everything in your life is fine, why do you think you wanted to end it?

I don't know. I guess I was just overreacting, because nothing in my life is really that bad.

Ally, you don't have to downplay the struggles you face in your life. Even though your issues may not seem like a big deal to some, they make up a part of your life. They are things you have to face and deal with every day. It's like when you fall in love. To the world, the person you love is just that, a single person. But to you, that person is everything. Just because other people have experienced horrific things in life, doesn't mean that your issues, your traumas, are any less significant.

I met with Vivian once a week for months, but that first conversation is what sticks with me the most. During our following sessions, we talked about my family, my parents, my siblings, and my role within the family. We talked about how I felt like I needed to be the person holding my entire family unit together, but that I had only just turned 16 years old, I was still very much a child. I'd been worrying about serious adult issues for years, like our home being foreclosed on, my sick little sister, and my parent's rocky relationship. She reminded me that it wasn't my responsibility to be the support system for my mom. Vivian urged me to think about how I was taking care of myself. "*I know you love your family, but when do you get to take care of Ally?*"

There were things I should have opened up about and talked with my therapist about like being groomed by an older man, my pre-mature involvement in sexual activity, experimenting with drugs, my nightmares, lack of self-worth, my boundless need for validation, and the anger that I still felt for failing at my suicide attempt. Maybe that would have helped me heal. But I just wanted to tie up the loose ends, box things up, and shove them someplace deep so we could all move past it. So, I put on a happy face. I smiled, said the right things, did the right things, and acted the right way. Eventually, I graduated from therapy, passing with flying colors.

I feel like it was shoved down my throat, that suicide was not an option. But if suicide was not an option, and I still didn't want to live, then there I was, stuck going through the motions of daily life on autopilot. I was numb inside, with no will to live, and no ambitions or dreams for the future. I didn't get excited or feel passionate about anything. Even my love for ballet was dwindling. I just kept doing it because, honestly, I didn't even know who I was without ballet as my identity. Every morning, I woke up just trying to get through enough of the day so that I could go back to bed.

I thought about trying to end my life again, I was sure I could have come up with a more fool proof plan. On the other hand, I was afraid of failing for a second time. However, there was something in my heart and gut that got triggered when I would brush my teeth. The mint of the peppermint patty that was supposed to be my last sweet treat before I said goodbye to this world still lingered. For years, the peppermint flavor of toothpaste when I brushed my teeth triggered a fear inside of me. Like I might accidentally try to kill myself, even if I wasn't intending to. I wasn't safe from myself. Not yet.

By all accounts, I had recovered and was thriving. *We gave more hugs.* That was the title of an article that Dad wrote, which was published in a magazine featuring suicide prevention stories. I literally rolled my eyes when my mom showed me the publication. In his article, he talked about how after my attempt, my family came together as a unit to make me feel more loved and included. Giving more hugs and planning more family activities: trips to the zoo, hiking, bowling, which is all true. My dad especially went out of his way again to spend more time with me. Teaching me how to drive and taking me to the bookstore. I treasured the time we got together. But it wasn't healing at all. If anything, I was angry.

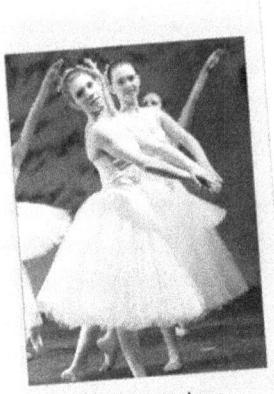

Playing my part as a
happy ballerina

If I thought that my family was my entire world before my attempt, they were now determined to be my entire universe. My world shrank to the size of our house. I wasn't allowed out for any reason without one of my parents. They even monitored the type of music I listened to. I lost whatever sense of self identity I had left. They claimed it was all so I could heal without distraction. But to me, it felt like they were trying to force me back into the mold of the old Ally, the one they remembered before everything had fallen apart. I played along, allowing them to believe that everything was okay. I got better at suppressing the darkness in front of others and playing the part of the happy family-oriented girl who loved ballet.

When my dad was 40 years old, he got his first tattoo —a serene Buddha etched beautifully on the inside of his forearm. *Remember, I was raised Buddhist and grew up going to the temple.* I was only about 8 at the time, but I thought his tattoo was beautiful—a true work of art. From that moment, I knew that one day I wanted to adorn my own skin with meaningful symbols. As a teenager, I started curating a digital gallery of tattoo designs I loved. The only problem was that I wasn't old enough. I didn't think I would make it to the age where I could make those decisions about my own body.

I've always loved to read, books were my sanctuary, worlds where I could escape from my reality. One of the things my dad and I would do together is go to Barnes & Noble. Dad would order a cup of coffee and meander through the music section, while I roamed the aisles, selecting a few books to lose myself in. Sometime *AA (After Attempt),* we went to Barnes & Noble, I picked out a book or two for my next *healthy escape.* As we went to the register, we passed that area of candies, knickknacks, and gift shop trinkets, and a notebook caught my eye. It had a bright blue butterfly on the cover next to the quote, *"When the caterpillar thought the world was over, she became a butterfly."*

The notebook spoke to my very existence. It was as if that quote was a message from the universe. In that moment, I saw myself as the caterpillar—lost, cocooned in darkness, yearning for transformation. The butterfly symbolizes hope, the possibility of emerging from despair into something vibrant and free. Maybe one day, I would become a butterfly.

I carried that image of the blue butterfly with me over the next few months. It became a symbol of hope and a reminder that there was beauty, life, and freedom in my future if I just held on. As my 17th birthday approached, I spent hours calling tattoo shops. I finally found one that would tattoo a minor with a signed parental permission form. And on my birthday, my dad took me to that dimly lit moody tattoo parlor. The shop was filled with gothic elegance and the steady hum of tattoo machines.

There was a burly man sitting at a drawing desk near the front of the shop. He welcomed us to the shop. I awkwardly presented him with a picture of a butterfly that I had printed out. He took the image and quickly drafted up a dainty butterfly stencil that he then permanently etched onto my back, after gaining my dad's signature of course. I sat through the process, each needle prick, a reminder that I was still alive, and would forever represent that quote from the notebook in Barnes & Noble.

Mom was pissed about the tattoo. *AA*, my relationship with my mom began to unravel. We no longer had the same close bond that we did before. Perhaps it was because she was still nursing the wounds left by my lies and deceit, the trust we had built over years had been shattered by my actions. On my end I resented all the freedoms that were taken away and the restrictions that had been put in place. I still helped her when she needed it—taking care of my siblings and assisting with photography jobs. But these acts of service felt hollow, tainted by a sense of obligation rather than genuine desire to be helpful.

No matter how closely my parents watched me, keeping me tightly under lock and key, I didn't stop finding ways to get into trouble. Whether it was sneaking out or sneaking people into the guest house in the backyard, I always managed to find a way. Desperate for validation I even resorted to online chat groups, websites that definitely weren't meant for girls under 18. I got a little more creative and got caught far less frequently.

When I was 18, my parents decided to move to Florida for my dad's work. I was petrified of change and had no desire to make such a big move across the country. How did I tell my parents that I was not going with them? That I refused to leave everything I have ever known in life? I didn't. I couldn't. I was so used to supporting my family that I had absolutely no idea how to advocate for myself or express my wants, needs, and desires in a mature adult manner.

My mom left with my sister to start setting up their new house in Miami. Without telling anyone, I quietly packed up all of my things, left a note on the desk in my dad's home office while he was at work, and moved out of our home and into my own apartment there in Phoenix. Breaking my family's heart, once again. I didn't even give them my new address. The first few months in my new place were great. I made new friends, I started partying, and it felt amazing to be an independent adult. I started picking up modeling gigs for extra cash and was proud that I was doing it. I was making it on my own.

All of my new-found friends were older than I was, which meant I had a steady supply of booze whenever I wanted it. *Jack and Coke, please.* Obviously, this was beyond dangerous for an unstable teen with a pit of darkness lurking inside. Drinking every night wasn't as fun as it had been at first, and I started scaring myself. The thoughts and dreams of killing myself became more and more frequent; the darkness got darker and louder than ever. Every day became a struggle with myself. Rather than succumbing to another suicide attempt, I begrudgingly made the decision to follow my parents to Florida for a fresh start.

When I got to Florida, everything was new. I no longer had my go-to connections for emotionless hookups and other bad decisions, so I turned all of my attention to my modeling career.

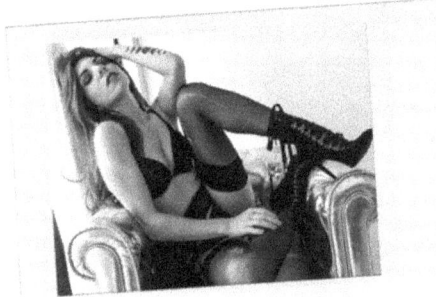

Being only 5 ft tall, I never thought it was possible to model. But I guess there are some exceptions if you have bright red hair and freckles, and I'd always been a performer. Because I'd spent years as the test subject of my mom's photography, I was pretty comfortable in front of the camera. As a young woman looking to get into modeling, Miami was definitely a good place to be. I met hair stylists and make-up artists who would doll me up before a photoshoot. The goal was always to make me look older, more mature. Most shoots had me posing in lingerie and high heels. In those pictures, I may have looked confident, but on the inside, I was still the self-conscious little girl who needed attention, love, and acceptance. I envied the woman in those photographs- she was someone I still didn't think I could ever be.

Friendly Neighborhood Walgreens Girl

I'd been working at Walgreens in the cosmetic department back in Arizona, so when I moved to Florida, it was easy for me to transfer to a new location in Miami Beach.

Even though I was just transferring stores, my new position at Walgreens felt both familiar and foreign. This was particularly apparent with my manager, Felipe, whose thick Spanish accent made his English nearly impossible to understand.

The computer systems and layout were almost the same but somehow also incredibly different. My first time on the register was stressful. I couldn't ask for help because even if I did, I wouldn't be able to understand the answer I got. I ended up pushing random buttons, trying to get the register to do what I needed it to do while the line of customers continued to get longer and longer. I was stressed and on the verge of tears. This new job was just the icing on the cake of how much I hated my life. I couldn't stand Miami: I didn't like the intense humidity, living with my parents again sucked, and now this!

Then this guy, a few customers deep waiting in line, startled to heckle me. *"What's taking so long?"* he laughed *"Why are you going so slow? Look at the line…"* His playful teasing, while it might have seemed cruel to onlookers, was exactly what I needed. It cut through my stress and added a flicker of amusement. Even causing me to smile for the first time that day, maybe even that week, that month.

When I got the chance, I finally looked up at the man who was poking fun at me. He was tall with long brown hair that went down to his waist, which was messily pulled back into a ponytail. The man's beard was nearly half as long as his hair cascading down to his chest. He wore a faded Harley Davidson hat backward on his head. He had large, gauged ears, piercings on his bottom lips, and several crappy-looking tattoos. His clothes were stained and dirty. His hands were calloused and filthy. At first glance, some might even say this man looked homeless. But when I looked at him, all I noticed were his gray-blue eyes and his friendly smile as he remarked casually, *"You're new here."* With that breaking of the ice, he made me forget all the stress I had experienced earlier that day.

"Yeah, I just moved to Florida."

I was starting to feel like this day would turn around until the man placed a case of beer on the counter of my register.

My heart sank. I sheepishly muttered.

"I'm only 19, I can't legally sell alcohol. I'll have to call my manager to help ring you up."

"Manager to the front," I squeaked over the loud intercom.

I waited a minute, then two, and no one came.

I laughed nervously as I stood there waiting for someone to relieve me of this awkward situation. Thankfully the bearded man was patient and understanding, as he welcomed me to Miami Beach. He told me he was a motorcycle mechanic, which I guess explained the grease-covered hands and oil-stained clothes. *So maybe he's not homeless after all.*

Since he was a mechanic, I thought maybe he would have connections to help me get a car, since I'd sold my old lemon in Arizona before I moved. I batted my eyes and asked him if he'd be able to help me out. He said absolutely and gave me his business card.

Luckily, after the third or fourth time of practically begging my manager over the intercom to come to my register, Felipe finally showed up. The patient man, whose business card stated his name to be Donny, could pay for his beer and leave.

I wasn't sure I would ever see him again, let alone that he would make good on his promise to help me find a car I could afford. Never in a million years would I have guessed that the man who just left the store would one day be my husband and father of my two kids.

Donny came back to Walgreens every day after he got off work. I always knew it was him pulling up to the front of the store because I could hear and recognize the loud rumble of his motorcycle. He came in to buy a pack of cigarettes from my register (because I was old enough to actually sell those), or sometimes he bought a 50-cent pack of peanuts just to pester me. He left me little notes like,

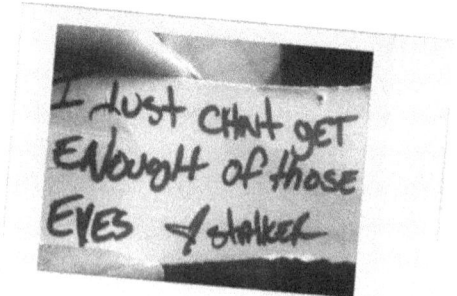

"I just can't get enough of those eyes - Stalker."

He asked me out a couple of times, but I just laughed and told him he was too old for me. *"Too old!"* he exclaimed. *"I'm only 26."*

But I just shook my head. Even if he wasn't 7 years older than me, I definitely wasn't into someone who DJ'ed at nightclubs on the weekends, got belligerently drunk, and had girls hanging on him each night. What can I say, when he wasn't covered, head to toe in grease and oil from work, he was quite the catch.

But Donny was persistent. He even found out when I took my lunch break and would come to sit with me outside of Walgreens. Sometimes, we shared a bag of chips as a snack. It was nice to have someone to pass the time with, but I definitely didn't think this was someone I could ever fall in love with.

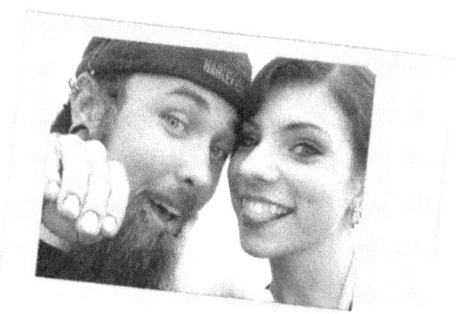

That's the thing about love. It can sneak up on you. He wore down the walls I'd put up around my heart, and I eventually agreed to spend time with him outside of work. For our first date, we met at the beach. He rode up on his motorcycle and I ran over to give him a kiss. In doing so, I clumsily burnt my leg on his scorching hot exhaust pipe. *Yes, I still have the scar today.* We walked on the beach, and eventually sat on a bench under a streetlamp, and talked for hours until well after the sun went down. We spoke about family, friends, life, and favorite foods. . . everything. Donny was the first person I'd met who made me feel as though I could be myself- my real self without hiding or editing out parts of who I was. I didn't have to try hard, fake a smile, or push to gain his attention. He genuinely liked me for who I was.

Falling in love was crazy and unexpected, but it felt natural. He was fun to be around. Being near him and becoming involved in each other's lives took my mind off the darkness inside and helped me adjust to life in Florida. In an interesting way, our lives just fit together. Being together was easy. Despite our outward differences, we connected on a deeper level— both of us carried scars from our respective pasts, and we just sort of accepted each other. It wasn't an adoring puppy love like I had felt in the past. It wasn't the whirlwind romance of fairy tales or the overwhelming butterflies of infatuation. Instead, it was a gradual realization—a feeling of comfort, companionship, and mutual support that grew stronger with each passing day. He became someone that I truly cared about, someone who I wanted to see succeed in life. I was only 19, but I knew that he was someone I wanted to build a life with. Sleeping next to him, my nightmares went away. A true testament to how much love can heal. Donny quickly became much more than just a chapter in my story. No matter what happened, we were partners and committed to working through things together.

A year into our relationship, I got pregnant. When I was 20 years old the idea of becoming a mom was absolutely terrifying. Donny was definitely not ready to settle down and become a father either. We were both still partying and enjoying life. We weren't ready to give up the drunken nights (okay, mornings) stumbling home after his DJ sets. Despite all that, a little voice inside my head kept saying that everything was going to be okay. Maybe it was hormones, maybe it was fate talking, but I already loved that little bean growing inside of me. I wanted to be his momma, no matter what sort of changes needed to happen. Donny felt the same, so we made the decision to move from our studio efficiency into a bigger one-bedroom apartment on the beach rather than purchasing a car with the money we'd saved up. We both stopped partying, opting to stay home and play video games together instead of going out.

When I told my parents I was pregnant, their reaction was a far cry from the supportive response I had hoped for. They were not just disappointed; they were visibly upset and worried. They had never been fond of Donny, the older guy who partied too much, and the news of my pregnancy only seemed to intensify their disdain. At 20 years old, I was already feeling overwhelmed by the situation, and their reaction made me feel like a little girl who was once again caught doing something wrong. I wanted to be happy and excited about this new chapter in my life, but I was held back by many of the same things that led to my suicide attempt. The negative opinions of others, combined with my parent's disapproval and my own insecurities, made it feel like my pregnancy was something to be hidden away rather than celebrated.

I actually found a surprising source of support from the regular customers while at work. Everyone knew the friendly redheaded girl who worked at the neighborhood Walgreens. Being bubbly and talkative, (*once I settled into Miami life*), I became quite acquainted with the locals. When they learned about my pregnancy, they were so sweet and encouraging, proclaiming that I was going to be a great mother. This was the response I wished would have come from my loved ones. As these regulars came into the store to pick up medicine from the pharmacy or to grab some snacks on the way home, they eagerly asked for updates and requested to see ultrasound pictures. When I shared the news that I was having a boy, they went out of their way to help. They brought gently used baby clothes that their own children had outgrown, gifted me essential baby supplies, and even gave me gift cards to support my growing family.

However, not everyone was so supportive. Working at Walgreens while my belly was growing increasingly noticeable felt like an invitation for strangers to voice unsolicited opinions. Some would make offhand remarks like, *"Having a baby so young means you'll always be relying on food stamps,"* or questioning whether my baby's father would actually stick around. Each comment felt like a personal attack, cutting through my already fragile sense of self-worth.

I was determined to push through the negativity though. I chose to be happy about my little boy and started to get more and more excited about his arrival. I washed all of his clothes, assembled his bed, and rearranged our bedroom to fit his crib next to where I slept. I took lots of pictures and tried to document my pregnancy well.

My mom took some maternity pictures for me. I didn't have a car at the time, so she drove me to the store to purchase a stroller and car seat with the gift cards I had received. It was nice to spend time together, especially since we didn't get much of it after I moved out of the family home and in with Donny. Unfortunately, this time together still didn't bridge the distance that seemed to stretch between us. I guess I thought being pregnant with my first child would look a little different. I thought back on all the time I spent rubbing her shoulders, back, and feet to make her feel as comfortable as possible when she was on bed rest with my youngest brother. I had always imagined that if I were ever pregnant, we'd share that same deep connection and nurturing bond. Yet, as I prepared for my own baby, I felt like I was still in trouble with her, and this was just another way I was continuing to disappoint my family.

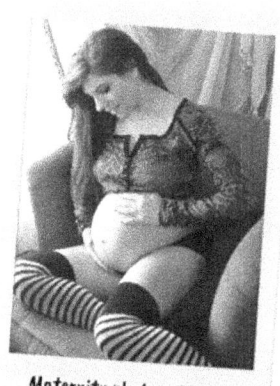

Maternity photos with our first baby

When it came down to those last month of pregnancy, I had to see my OB weekly. At one of those last appointments, the doctor sat me down for a serious discussion about the options for delivery: the benefits and risks of a natural birth versus a C-section. As I listened, my mind whirled with fear. The thought of being cut open and undergoing major surgery was terrifying. Yet, the prospect of enduring hours of intense, painful labor with no one to truly support me felt even more daunting.

Donny, who had little knowledge about childbirth, wouldn't know what to do in that situation. Even though I knew my mom would come to the delivery if I asked, I was still worried she wouldn't be able to comfort me in the way I needed in those raw and vulnerable moments of labor. I felt overwhelmed, lonely, and scared.

As the doctor laid out both options, he made it really seem like a cesarean would be the best option for the baby, but ultimately it was my choice. I decided to go with an elective C-section. It felt like the safest bet and gave me a bit of control over the situation. Yet, I couldn't help feeling like I took the easy way out. I was faced with troubling thoughts like, if I wasn't willing to face the pain and trials of labor and childbirth, maybe I wasn't ready to be a mother.

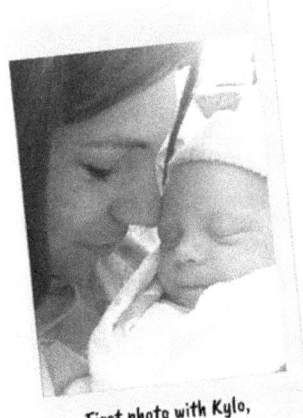

First photo with Kylo,
love at first sight

When our son, Kylo, was born, it was love at first sight. I couldn't believe that I was able to bring something so beautiful into this world. The birth of a child is both a challenging and rewarding experience for a mother, no matter how it happens. Although I was tired and dazed from the pain medication, due to the c-section, it didn't stop me from feeling blissful as a new mom. The act of motherhood seemed so natural to me. Baby snuggles, feeding, and diaper changes gave me little glimmers of happiness.

I loved that little baby curled up on my chest, but Kylo was a challenging baby. Sometimes he would cry and cry long into the night, no matter how much nursing, burping, swaddling, and rocking I did. *What was I doing wrong? I read all the books, and I helped take care of my siblings growing up, but nothing could have prepared me for those early days of motherhood.* Those sleepless nights started to add up. Combine that physical and emotional exhaustion with the fact that I needed to return back to work at Walgreens only six weeks after giving birth, and my initial euphoria of motherhood quickly faded. Most of the new friends I'd made in Miami were still in their party phase and didn't want to spend time hanging out in my apartment with a wailing baby. I felt isolated and lonely like no one understood what I was going through.

My mom watched Kylo most days while Donny and I were working. I saw how well she took care of him, and how easily she could calm him down when he would go into one of his crying fits. I really felt that she was a much better mother than I ever could be. I was overwhelmed with feelings of inadequacy. Not only was I not being a good enough mom, but I was also failing as a homemaker. I'd get off work, pick up the baby, and come home to piles of laundry, dishes, and endless chores that needed to be done. I was spiraling… I was convinced that everyone would be better off if I weren't around, but I also knew I couldn't leave my son without a mom.

Postpartum can be a difficult time for a lot of women. For me, postpartum depression made everything feel even more unmanageable, especially when I sensed that familiar tug of the darkness. No one would ever have known that I was struggling. I had been practicing masking my true feelings, thoughts, and emotions for far too long. I was so good at portraying the joyous new mommy. That's what makes suicidal ideation so scary. You never know who is carrying those dark thoughts. Your sister, your best friend, or your co-worker may be concealing mental health concerns with a smile or humor.

I tried not to be home alone very often. On my days off, I went on long walks with the baby, tried to meet up with new mom friends, and went back to modeling as soon as I got my "body" back. But it still didn't make the deep-rooted feelings of inadequacy go away.

Stupid, broken, Ally. I had everything that most little girls dream of as children. I had a partner who loved me unconditionally, giving me all the love and attention I could ever need or want. I had a beautiful baby boy who deserved a happy and attentive mother. I had a roof over my head, food in my belly, and was physically healthy…yet I still couldn't keep the darkness away.

So, I started bargaining with myself. *Ally, if you just stay alive until you're done breastfeeding, then your son won't need you anymore, and then you can kill yourself.*

Okay, okay, okay. If you can just get to his first birthday, then he won't need you anymore…

At first, it was just the occasional thought:

While walking to work: *What if I accidentally stepped out into oncoming traffic?*

On my days off, during my long walks, *what if I went to the beach and started swimming until my arms and legs gave out?*

Then, these thoughts started happening more frequently. And I got to a place where I was fantasizing more about death than life.

Minty toothpaste started to trigger me again. I was literally scared of myself; I was once again afraid of what I knew I was capable of.

I knew that if something didn't change, I would not see my son grow up and would not be able to grow old with Donny. I loved my family; I loved the little life I was living. But I still didn't love myself. All I saw in the mirror was the darkness I was suppressing.

I needed something to live for outside of the endless laundry, a job I hated, and the thankless tasks that come with motherhood.

I needed something to drive me forward.

I needed something to be passionate about.

I needed a goal.

 # 26.2

Instead of buying a convertible, my dad decided to run his first marathon when he hit his so-called "mid-life crisis."

For months, he'd juggle workdays with treadmill runs at the gym, even dedicating Saturday mornings to pounding the pavement. I couldn't fathom the appeal of waking up early on weekends just to run when I could lounge on the couch watching cartoons.

The day of his first race came.

I was woken up early by my parents, the sun wasn't even up. It was an unexpectedly cold winter day in Phoenix, Arizona; I was about 8 years old and wore one of my mom's Chicago Bears sweatshirts which, on my tiny body, was oversized, covering my hands and falling down below my knees. I had no idea what to expect.

Thousands of people lined the streets as waves of runners sped by. I looked through the legs of the people in front of me, hoping to glimpse my dad. I wiggled my way to the front of the crowd, and reached out my sleeve-covered hand, hoping that one of the runners might give me a high-five as they passed by.

The runners looked so tired, shoulders hunched forward, feet shuffling, flushed faces even though it was chilly outside... But as they passed, a few runners gave me a high five, and I offered them some words of encouragement *"Woo, keep going! You're doing great!"*

That little bit of positive reinforcement made their backs straighten, adding a little extra pep to their step, and put a smile on their faces. That's when it all came together for me as to why my dad had spent all that time preparing for this race. These people running were doing something tough. Something big! Something that took months of training. In my mind as a young child… what they were doing was something AMAZING. Something that mattered. I mean, look at the huge crowd of people who'd gotten up early on their weekend just to stand outside in the cold morning air, and cheer them on.

After countless high-fives and cheers, I finally saw my dad. He was devouring a handful of gummy bears (apparently, that's running fuel???). Although my dad was a sweaty mess, he had the biggest smile I had ever seen on his face. He gave us a quick hello and kept on trekking.

My mom, siblings, and I quickly got in the car and drove to the finish line, where we again found my dad in the crowd.

I hugged my dad. He had a medal around his neck and was eating a banana.

Wow... so you get gummy bears, high-fives, a banana, AND a medal?!?!?

Sign me up!!!!

So, at only 8 years old, while most of my classmates were dreaming about being astronauts, movie stars, or race car drivers, I decided that if I ever grew up, I would run a marathon.

The problem was... I hated running. And I wasn't any good at it.

This disdain was so prevalent that I actually got my ballet teacher to write a note saying I couldn't run the mile in high school because it would interfere with my dancing.

So, the idea of actually running 26.2 miles seemed like one of those dreams, you know the ones. *Sure, I'd love to go to Antarctica and see Emperor penguins. But the idea of dealing with that intense cold and paying the extremely expensive travel fees to see penguins that still need several yards of space, that no one's allowed to hug...* not something that will actually ever happen.

But life has a funny way of making things happen.

This memory suddenly hit me years later when I was all grown up, with a child of my own. That child happened to be napping in the other room, and I found myself in the kitchen, trying to hype myself up to do the dishes. Yet there I stood, with a pit in my stomach and a feeling of heaviness in my chest instead of a newfound enthusiasm for cleaning bottles. I opted to make another cup of coffee instead, probably the 4th one that day. Emotionally and physically exhausted, I sank to the floor with my coffee mug. I took long, deep gulps, even as I felt it burning my tongue and throat. I remember thinking, at least I was feeling something other than misery and helplessness.

There had to be more to life. There had to be something worth living for outside of my wifely and motherly duties. Sitting on the kitchen floor, nursing my cup of coffee, I mindlessly scrolled on the internet with a mixture of desperation and hopelessness. That's when I stumbled across an ad for the Miami Marathon.

A marathon…

My mind flickered back to my dad proudly wearing his marathon medal.

I could get a medal.

There is no award for washing the most loads of laundry in a day, no gold star for cooking your family dinner every night, no pats on the back for waking up with a crying baby… Nope.

But I could get a medal for running a marathon.

I could get a medal and recognition for being part of the 1% of the world that runs 26.2 miles.

At that moment, I made a silent vow. I would cross the finish line of a marathon before I died. I could not fall victim to my darkness before I crossed this one thing off my bucket list.

Sure, looking back now, I realize that I was once again bargaining with myself. But, for the first time in a very long time, I had a goal—a personal goal. There was something to look forward to and something to drive me forward. It wasn't just a goal; it became my lifeline, a glimmer of hope amidst the shadows that nearly consumed my life.

That next weekend, I set my alarm for early in the morning, long before my husband and son would wake up. I put on a pair of cheap, no brand-name sneakers, and went out the front door for my very first run. I'd barely made it to the end of the street before I was huffing and puffing. When I stopped to catch my breath and turned around, I could still see my mailbox. Instead of beating myself up for being so out of shape, I focused on the fact that I'd run a whole 100 yards. This first little run was a huge turning point for me. It was alright that I was going to have to work to achieve this goal. I knew that tomorrow, I was going to get better, faster, and run further. For the first time that I could recall, I focused on my potential instead of dwelling on all of my shortcomings or giving in to the darkness.

I was sort of embarrassed by my goal to run a marathon. I was terrified to tell anyone and was even afraid to tell Donny that I wanted to start running. I knew that if he thought it was a stupid idea, I would be absolutely crushed. Looking back, I know this was a silly fear because that's one of the things I love most about our relationship. Donny and I have always been extremely supportive of each other in every aspect of our lives, no matter how crazy a goal or dream may seem at first.

When I finally sheepishly told him that I wanted to run a marathon, Donny responded with unwavering support. *"What do you need to accomplish this goal?"* I told him I could really use a pair of actual running shoes since the sneakers I was currently wearing were really hurting my feet.

At the time, we were young and broke. So broke that in the days before payday Donny and I would split our last $10 bill so we could both at least buy a bag of chips for lunch. The idea of spending $120+ dollars on a pair of shoes for a hobby that I may or may not actually follow through with was insane. But Donny has always supported me in any way he can. He took me to Dick's Sporting Goods the same night that I confessed my goal of completing a marathon. Neither of us knew much about running shoes, and the store staff weren't much help. In the end, I chose a pair of fairly random shoes in my favorite shade of pinkish magenta, simply because that was my favorite color - not because those were the best shoes for my feet and stride.

I was absolutely elated to have my very first pair of running shoes. Those bright pinkish magenta shoes meant more than our having to cut down on groceries for a while. *Who doesn't like a month's worth of butter noodles?* Those shoes meant that Donny believed in me, that he supported me. Every time I laced them up, I was committing to achieving my crazy goal. I was actually going to run a marathon, no matter how hard it would be.

I was excited to start training officially.

I didn't know how I would get in my training runs. Kylo, my little companion in life, was with me nearly every waking moment when I wasn't working at my barely above minimum wage job. My husband worked long hours during the week, so running before or after his 12-hour days was less than ideal. Maybe I could run on the weekends when he was home to watch the little one? As little as I knew about running, I did know from watching my dad train all those years before that I needed to run more than just once or twice a week if I wanted to complete a marathon.

I went into problem-solving mode. There was a gym about a mile and a half away from my house. This LA Fitness had an option to include an hour of childcare a day while members used the gym. "*Okay, if I am really smart with my money, I can get a gym membership and take Kylo to the kid care. But then came the logistical hurdle—how would I even get to the gym?*"

At the time, Donny had his motorcycle, but we didn't own any other vehicle. Things were extremely tight financially, and I had always been able to either walk or use public transit in Miami. But there was no bus or trolly routes from my home to the gym. Sure, I did have a stroller, but not one designed for running. Attempting to jog with it risked either poor Kylo getting shaken baby syndrome or breaking a wheel. Yet, the stroller had been our trusty companion for daily errands, walks to the grocery store, and to the bank. Why not extend its use to walk to the gym? So, that's just what I did. Three to four times a week, I loaded Kylo into the stroller, braved the mile and a half trek to the gym, and checked him into the kid club, where I'd then deal with the guilt of him crying because he didn't want me to leave him. After finishing my run on the treadmill, I picked him back up and retraced our path, pushing the stroller back home.

Yes, it was time-consuming and exhausting, but I didn't even think twice about it. Instead, each journey to and from the gym became a testament to my determination to cross the finish line.

I had learned to be resourceful, leveraging every option available to me. I had learned to see challenges as opportunities, to find solutions.

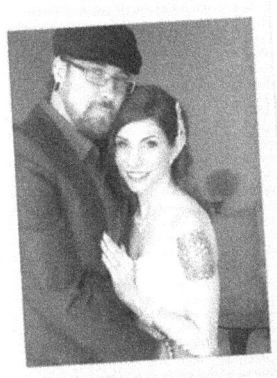

Mr & Mrs Robinson

During this time, Donny and I finally said our "I dos." *Who said it had to be love, marriage, and THEN the baby carriage?* We might have done things a little out of order, but it was the perfect timing for us. Donny proposed to me on the beach at sunrise, it felt so surreal! After years of feeling inadequate and unlovable, finally, someone that I cared for so deeply wanted to marry me?! It was a small ceremony with only immediate family present. After the vows, we celebrated by going to P.F. Chang's, I didn't even bother to change out of my wedding dress. The staff was shocked to see us come in, honored that we were sharing our big day with them, they even brought us free dessert. As a wedding gift, Donny purchased my entry into the Miami Marathon. Making my goal as official as we were.

I looked forward to my training runs. The moment I finished one workout, I was already looking forward to the next time I could lace up my running shoes. I was getting stronger and faster. Don't get me wrong, I made a lot of mistakes. Maybe even every mistake: I ran in the wrong kind of shoes, I ran too fast, I had terrible running form, I didn't follow a training plan, I never warmed up or cooled down. I read all the running blogs that laid out how to run a marathon and they all gave the same advice, which I ignored. Maybe I thought I was the exception to the rule, or maybe I was self-sabotaging.

When I went for a run, my goal was always to get done as quickly as possible. A lot of the reason why I cut down on anything that felt excessive, like warming up or stretching, was because I had so much guilt over leaving my now toddler in someone else's care or taking time away from my family. My identity now was tied to being a mom and a wife. I had to squeeze in the part of me that also really wanted to be a runner. Taking shortcuts and rushing the process is not advisable when it comes to running or training for a marathon, and ultimately led to my downfall as an athlete.

I built my mileage up to 10 miles. But after that first 10-mile run, I felt a stabbing pain on the side of my knee. I literally limped home and iced it. After a day or two of rest, my knee felt better. Thinking I was healed, I went out for a short run to test things out. Within a few short minutes, that sharp, stabbing pain stopped me in my tracks again.

After consulting Doctor Google, I concluded that it was my IT band flaring up. I still had months before the marathon, so I decided to give it a week or two of rest. But a week or two of rest led to a month or two of rest, and my motivation to run and train was completely gone.

The momentum of running had carried over into my professional life. I had moved on from Walgreens and started looking for better job opportunities. I got a job as a receptionist at a Spa and Fitness Center. With hard work I was able to quickly climb up the ladder to a management position. Of course, this was a much more demanding job, and I used that as an excuse. *I didn't have time to run!* I was working to better myself and my family's financial situation.

So much about me changed in the short time since I had started running and training for the marathon. It was as though I'd finally woken up from this zombie-like haze and started to actually live life. I woke up excited for the day and looked forward to the future. Because of my new management job, I was finally able to afford a car. I was getting healthier and happier. I even started enjoying motherhood a whole lot more because I had my own dreams and goals.

Even though I worked more outside of the home, I was able to spend more quality time with my husband and son. I wasn't just living on autopilot anymore; I was finally taking control of my life.

The date of the race was getting closer and closer. I knew I needed to start running and training again, but I was so afraid of my IT Band flaring up that I just avoided running altogether. As time moved on and the marathon was only six weeks away, I knew I needed to do something. That finish line, that medal, was keeping me alive… It was why my life was so drastically changing for the better.

I ran a very slow 3-mile run, and everything seemed okay. Great- I could start training again! But how? I started Googling. *"How to train for a marathon in 6 weeks."* Literally, every forum said it was stupid, impossible, and dangerous. But in my mind, I was still the exception. I started training my own way. Five weeks before the marathon, I attempted a 7-mile run. At about the halfway mark, I felt that familiar pain on the outside of my knee. According to my Google searches, IT Band Syndrome was painful but would (hopefully) unlikely cause long-term injury if I kept pushing through the pain.

So, that's what I did.

Four weeks out from the marathon, I ran 8 miles, three weeks out from the marathon, I made my second attempt at double digits. I knew this would be my last long run before the race. My knee hurt so bad that I had to fight to keep moving forward, limping more than running. But I finished. I knew from there I could taper down and focus on resting and recovering as much as possible so my IT Band would be in the best possible condition on race day. I figured I'd just end up limping the last few miles if things hadn't completely healed.

When people asked if I was running the marathon, I confidently told them I was just running the half marathon. That way, no one would know that I failed yet again if the worst possible scenario happened on race day, and I needed to stop at the halfway mark. I knew in my heart that I needed to finish the full marathon no matter what, even if for no other reason than to prove to myself that I could.

The evening before the race, my now husband, Donny, took me to IHOP to carb-load on pancakes. I love pancakes! However, when dinner was served, I couldn't stomach them. I was so nervous that I felt sick, and that night I couldn't sleep. I tossed and turned, checking the time every few minutes to make sure I hadn't missed my alarm. I tried to eat breakfast, but I couldn't manage more than a couple of bites. My hands physically shook as I tied up the laces of my running shoes. I tried to listen to music to take slow deep breaths, anything to calm my nerves. I had never experienced jitters like this before any modeling shoot or big performance as a dancer. Those things hadn't mattered to me the way this race did.

Donny, always my rock, held my hand as he drove me to the start line.

"You got this, babe," he reassured me as I got out of the car.

The Miami Marathon is a massive race: thousands of runners lined the streets, jam-packed into designated corrals. The atmosphere was electric with anticipation from the runners and the spectators alike. It had rained earlier in the morning, and the streets were wet. My pinkish-magenta shoes were soaked through before we even started. Despite the warmth, goosebumps prickled my skin as the National Anthem resonated through the crowd. Tears welled up in my eyes as a mixture of nerves and determination flooded my senses. This was it—the moment that had kept me alive for the past year. I had no idea what sort of pain and discomfort lay ahead of me, but I knew I would fight like hell to finish this race.

The horn blared, signaling the start of the race, and I started running. Initially, I felt pretty good. I had never experienced the adrenaline rush of running with a herd of fellow runners, and I was beyond excited. For the first few miles of the Miami Marathon route, the runners cross the Macarthur Causeway, a long bridge that runs along the port of Miami. It is quite the scenic way to view Miami as the sun rises and cruise ships in the port prepare for takeoff.

By Mile 7, my run had devolved into more of a limp. My IT Band was flared up and angry—like, really angry. Each step was a harsh reminder of my insufficient training. I tried to stop and stretch, but there was a 7-hour cut-off time to complete the race. I just felt like I was wasting time, time that I needed. I didn't want to run the whole damn race just to watch the race organizers pack up the finish line before I got there.

I tried to ignore the pain in my leg the best I could. Every time I came across a photographer taking pictures, I tried really hard to replace the grimace on my face with a big smile. *I was having the time of my life, right?* Most of my training for the marathon had been on a treadmill, pressed for time to finish so I could pick up my son from kid care. During the race I realized how enjoyable it was to run outside. All the things to see! I enjoyed the people watching, the great views Miami had to offer, and of course, it was fun to read the signs made by the spectators. I saw kids standing along the side of the race, cheering. I was reminded of my own experience watching my dad run his first marathon so many years before.

I missed my dad, I really wished he could have been there to support me. He'd moved back to Phoenix right after my wedding and couldn't make it back for the marathon. It was like the universe knew I was reminiscing about my dad, and the playlist I was listening to through my headphones started playing a song by his favorite band, *Guided by Voices.*

The first time I saw my husband during the race was around mile 11. I was so grateful to Donny for being there for me. It's amazing how much just seeing a loved one can boost your spirits, even temporarily. This was the farthest I had ever run. While I was in pain, it was no worse than I felt in training; I knew I could keep going. At the halfway mark, the race splits. Half marathoners go one way to head back toward the finish line, and full marathoners go the other way to keep the suffering going. Between the two paths, there's a huge barrier separating the two groups. I remember looking longingly at the half marathoners. They were within reach of the finish line. I could go that way. I really could. No one would think less of me. After all, I had told everyone that I was *"just"* doing the half marathon.

But in my head, quitting at 13 miles was NOT an option.

After I passed the split mark for the race, I started to feel this new pain in my shoe. My toes, specifically my toenails, felt like they were being slowly peeled off with pliers… probably because they were actually separating from the nailbed. I called my husband, *"Houston, we have a problem. I am pretty sure my toenails are falling off. Meet me as soon as you can."*

Donny met me around mile 18. I sat down in the grass on the side of the road and pulled off my shoe. My sock was soaked from running on the wet pavement, but also with my blood. Two of my toenails had huge angry blisters under them, causing them to hang loose and bloody at the end of my toes.

I held back the vomit that threatened to fill my mouth. I took the medical tape that my husband was carrying in my emergency bag and taped up my toes the best I could. Trying to put my shoe back was excruciatingly painful. It's like my shoes were two sizes too small. I had no idea that it was normal for feet to swell while running long distances. I was absolutely paying the price for not getting properly fitted for shoes, and not buying running shoes in the next size up. I felt like Cinderella's stepsisters trying to shove their feet into the glass slipper. *Honestly, at this point, running in glass slippers would have probably been more comfortable. Or maybe I should have been like Cinderella and ditched the shoes on the side of the road.* I jammed my shoe back on and kept going.

Every step made me want to cry. My bleeding toes radiated pain throughout my foot. My IT band seized up. I couldn't even bend my knee at this point. Maybe it was that mythical wall runners talk about hitting at some point in a long race, or my very evident lack of training. Whatever it was, I was way deep in the pain cave.

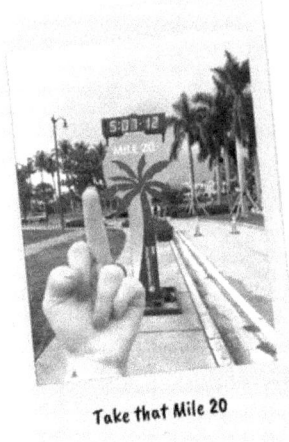

Take that Mile 20

I came up to the mile marker 20. I pulled out my phone and took a picture of me flashing the bird to the 20-mile mark, with the clock just ticking along. Those roadside race timers just kept reminding me that no matter how much pain I was in, I needed to get my butt into gear if I was going to avoid the cut-off. I sent the picture to Donny, hoping he would find some humor in it, and as I put my phone away, I attempted to start running again.

I was so far behind those who had trained properly for the race that there really wasn't anyone in front of me. At that point, no one was behind me either. As I ran with my limping leg, I occasionally passed another really struggling marathon participant. Thankfully, they were so caught up in their own struggle that they didn't even notice my crying. I kept whispering to myself, *"Quitting is not an option, quitting is not an option."*

I saw Donny again at Mile 22. I fell into his arms, and cried into his chest…

"This is NOT FUN! Why did I do this to myself?"

He dried my tears and laughed as he told me he would see me at the finish line. He was more confident than I was that I would finish this marathon.

I didn't want to leave my husband, my rock. I wished he would pick me up and carry me home. I wish he would have just told me that it was okay to quit. And that he was proud of me for even attempting.

But he didn't. He just sent me on my way.

The second I started to walk, well limp away from Donny, I knew I had just made a huge mistake. I wanted to quit—so badly. Please, just someone, end my misery, pull me out of the race, let me get picked up by the sweep bus, man. I'll even take a meteor falling out of the sky and crushing me.

Everything hurt so bad that it reminded me of that green hallway. When I'd been so exhausted, my weak legs, not strong enough to carry my body weight without leaning on a walker for support. All I'd wanted to do then was sit down and cry. But they wouldn't let me. The people in scrubs kept pushing me further down the hallway, towards the unknown, towards my future.

But I wasn't in that green hallway. I was participating in the Miami Marathon, and I had just run 23 fucking miles.

There was no one here to tell me what to do.

So, at mile 23, I sat on the curb and cried.

I had come so far but still felt so far away from finishing 26.2 miles.

I could quit——I could quit right now. I could call my husband to pick me up, walk away from the race, and no one would blame me. Some might even find it heroic for me to attempt a marathon.

I could quit.

But I know what it's like to quit.

I had tried to quit on life before, and I didn't want to feel like that again.

I don't want to live life walking around on autopilot like a damn zombie.

I want to dream big and chase those goals.

I want to feel that passion in my heart and that excitement for a new day.

I want to see my son grow up

I want to grow old with my husband.

Quitting was an option, but with every step towards the finish line I was choosing to keep moving forward, I was choosing to keep going, I was choosing life.

As I was contemplating all this, a volunteer at an aid station must have thought I was overheating. I can only assume she was trying to be helpful when she unexpectedly wrung a sponge full of icy cold water on the back of my neck. It was like a slap in the face, bringing me out of that green hallway and back to reality.

I stood up, gritted my teeth, and started moving toward the finish line.

With every step I took, I thought about the green hallway. I thought about struggling to walk in my hospital gown and socks, trying to hold up my weight on the walker. If I could make it down that hallway, I could finish this race. I choose to keep going. I choose life.

So, I ran. No matter how blinding the pain became, I kept pushing forward.

The marathon path narrowed, and metal fences corralled the runners to the finish line.

I had imagined crossing the finish line hundreds of times throughout the past year.

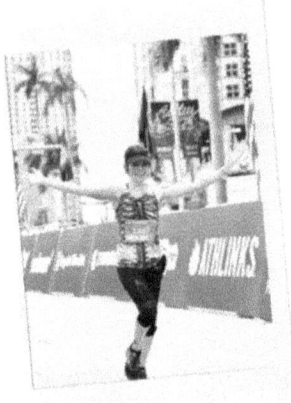

Flying to the Finish

Throwing out my arms like a human airplane and flying into the finish line.

I felt my arms extend out from my sides.

This was really happening!

I was flying to the finish line!

Tears again poured down my face. *But this time not from pain...*

I crossed that finish line. My husband was there cheering me on, and I felt something I had never felt before.

PRIDE.

For once in my life, I felt PROUD of myself.

I did this! I didn't give up.

I didn't quit.

I ran a marathon.

I posted on Facebook that night…

"One small step for women… One giant leap for these little legs."

Through tears and laughter, pain, and triumph, I had not just completed a marathon——I had conquered my fears, rediscovered my strength, and found something that lit a fire within me.

I didn't find a reason worth living. I created it.

Ally Robinson

Becoming Coach Ally

Before my IT Band had even started to recover, my toenails had grown back, or I could walk normally without a limp, I was already thinking about my next race. I needed to line up my next goal, and maybe the one after that, too! Turns out, the finish line at the Miami Marathon wasn't an endpoint but the gateway to a new beginning, a fresh chapter in my journey as a runner and in my life—something that I now call the *Endless Race*.

This time, I decided to approach it differently. I had to be smarter and more deliberate. I joined a local running group, immersing myself in a community of like-minded individuals who shared my passion. I went to an actual running store and got fitted properly, by a professional, for a new pair of running shoes that worked for my feet. With the extra money I made from my management job, I also hired a running coach to guide me on this path. It was time to set aside the rebellious ways that had been holding me back and focus on building a stronger foundation… I was all in.

My coach taught me the importance of proper running form and introduced me to a series of corrective exercises designed to address my knocked knees and overpronation. I had known for a long time that I had knocked knees. What I didn't know is that overpronation, or walking/running on the inside of my foot, caused my arches to cave in and exacerbated my knocked knees. My coach taught me that strengthening my glutes and hips would help correct the angle of my knees. With those muscles strengthened, my running form improved, which helped prevent future IT band syndrome flare-ups. After feeling the pain relief and realizing the power of small changes, I became almost obsessed with fine-tuning every aspect of my training.

I started keeping a journal with all the data collected from my runs, keeping track of what shoes worked best for which types of runs, what time of day I had the most energy, and what nutrition made me perform my best. After a few months of adjusting which exercises I did and prioritizing form during those exercises, along with a strategic running plan I saw significant improvement in my speed and endurance.

A really valuable lesson I learned from working with my coach was how to be open and honest about how I am feeling physically and mentally. After years of masking, it was a challenge to be open about the daily struggles of a runner. Admitting that I was exhausted due to insufficient sleep, overwhelmed by work stress, or grappling with soreness in my calf or an upset stomach after a run was something I found incredibly challenging.

By acknowledging these issues, rather than brushing them aside or trying to push through them, I began to see a remarkable change in my approach to training and my overall well-being. It became clear that the journey wasn't just about pushing my physical limits; it was about understanding and addressing the underlying factors that affected my performance and daily life. I didn't have to navigate all this alone. By being open and honest about how I was feeling, I could get the support I needed to find solutions to my problems and continue to improve.

The progress I saw wasn't just physical; it was empowering. I started running in local races, which there are a ton of in Miami. It seemed like every couple of weeks, I was either placing in the top 3 of my age group or getting a new PR (*Personal Record*). These victories, small as they might seem, created giant leaps in my confidence. Running and training strategically wasn't just about moving faster——it was about unlocking a potential within myself that I hadn't realized I had lying dormant within me.

At this point, I was completely different from the year prior, and several of the local moms I knew with kids about the same age as my son began to take notice. They saw a happier, healthier version of me. When they asked about my secret, I shrugged my shoulders. *"Uh, I don't know. I just run."* So, I invited them to come on a run with me. The women looked at me like I was crazy. Running was something none of them had even considered. They did see the positive change in me, though, and were grappling with their own stresses of motherhood, and still trying to lose the baby weight. Hesitantly, a few women agreed to meet at the beach the next weekend for a run. We started slowly, I talked to them about pacing, how to build up endurance, and controlling their breathing. I was simply passing on the wisdom that I had gained from experience, in the running groups I had joined, and that my running coach had given me.

The women actually enjoyed the runs! With the information and guidance, I was passing on to them, they improved pretty quickly, experiencing all the wonderful benefits that I had recently experienced myself. Sharing my newfound love for running with others gave me even more fulfillment and purpose.

As much as I loved my new life, being a manager was exhausting! Especially since I'd just switched jobs again to a higher-paying salaried position, running a beauty salon. The young receptionists often called out, leaving me to cover double shifts at the front desk while also keeping inventory, managing staff, and setting up interviews. Clients could be overly demanding, entitled, and presumptuous even if everything else was running smoothly. Then when I was able to be at home, I was always on call. My mind was still at work when I wanted to be fully present with my family.

Running became my sanctuary, a way to de-stress, reclaim some peace, and quiet my mind. Yet, even as I thrived, I couldn't shake the feeling that I was missing out on precious moments with my son. The long hours and demanding work schedule had me in survival mode, juggling all these responsibilities. Why did I still feel like I was just scraping by, that I could do more for both myself and my family?

I went to the gym after work one day to get in a quick workout before I needed to pick up my son from preschool. I would have rather been running, but at this point, I knew how important strength training was to my overall running goals. I put on my headphones and started to listen to an audiobook to get my mind off of the squats and lunges I had on my training plan for that day. I was listening to Rachel Hollis's book *Girl, Wash Your Face*. As I listened to Rachel's story about starting and growing her business as a mom, I was inspired. I heard that little voice in my head, *"Could I do that? Could I turn my love for running into a career? Those women that I have been running with, would they actually be willing to pay me for my expertise?"*

Sitting in the locker room of the gym, I began exploring what I needed to do, and what actions I should take in order to turn that little voice into a plan. I researched the cost and time commitment of obtaining coaching and personal training certifications. Ideas and possibilities buzzed in my head. When my husband got home that night, I presented him with the idea of returning to school to become a running coach. He looked at me with a bit of disbelief; I had just worked for months to gain the experience I needed to move into my current management position I was in. Once the initial shock quickly wore off, as always, he wholeheartedly believed in me. That night, before I could second my plans, he pulled out the credit card and made the first payment for my first class. This payment was just one of the many ways he helped me towards my newfound dream of becoming a certified personal trainer and running coach. I never needed his permission or approval to pursue my personal or professional goals, but it felt so good to have his support. This was a life changing decision, and we were going to need to share this goal and work as a team to make it through the transition period.

That next season of life was extremely challenging, but not like the challenges I had in the past. I had work, school, my son Kylo, and still somehow needed to maintain my own training runs. Not to mention the fact that we only had one car at the time, which increased the logistical challenges because I was driving my husband to and from work when his motorcycle was out of commission or on rainy days. Amidst this chaos, I felt a thrilling buzz of energy, similar to the excitement I felt before the start of my first marathon. My life was once again changing.

Growing up, I was never a good student, barely passing classes, neglecting homework, and often failing tests. Because I nearly flunked out of school. I carried the idea that I was dumb. Turns out I was just bored of school and disinterested in classes I saw no need for. Everything shifted now that I was studying a subject I was and am still really interested in. Learning all about anatomy, new training strategies, and how to actually coach other people was so exciting. I even made flashcards to study on the go. When I passed my certification exams on the first attempt, it was a revelation. I was smarter and more capable than I had ever given myself credit for.

The first time I actually confessed to someone other than my husband that I was pursuing a career as a personal trainer and running coach was one afternoon when I went to a salon to get my hair cut. With all my new life changes, I felt like I needed to make a change in my appearance as well. My waist-length red hair had been a part of my identity for so long, whether it was neatly tied up into a bun for ballet or styled for a photo shoot. I wanted something fresh, something not so sweaty when I ran, something that signaled a new chapter in my life. So, I decided to cut my waist-long hair into a short bob, donating over 10 inches of hair.

Sitting in that salon chair, I felt a mix of excitement and nervousness. When the stylist politely asked me what it was that I did for a living, my heart skipped a beat. I sheepishly confessed, "*I am a running coach.*" I held my breath, petrified that he was going to call me out. *You don't look like a coach, How many clients do you have? How long have you been coaching?* I braced myself for a flood of questions that would expose me as a fraud. Instead, he simply responded with, "*Cool.*"

It was such a simple word, but it carried so much weight. It felt like a small victory, a moment of validation that I needed. With that one word, he confirmed that I could own my new title of Coach Ally.

Those women I had started running with on the weekends, sharing my tips, tricks, and insights, became my first official paying clients. They enthusiastically gave me money in exchange for continuing to coach them on their journey. It was surreal. Here were these amazing women who believed in me, trusted me to guide them, and were willing to invest in my coaching.

Initially, I felt a massive wave of imposter syndrome. I was convinced someone would call me out or question my credentials. I had only been running for a couple of years at this point. I wasn't the fastest runner, I wasn't a track star, and I certainly wasn't an Olympic athlete. *Did I really have what it took to be a great coach?*

Every time I met with a new client or attended a running event, those doubts crept in. I would look around at other coaches, their impressive resumes, and their confident demeanors, and I felt like I didn't belong. It was exhausting, constantly battling with my own insecurities.

Over time, I started to see things differently. I've learned that it's okay to have doubts, but it's important not to let them control you. I realized that being a great coach isn't about being the fastest or born with great athletic ability. It's about passion, dedication, and the genuine desire to help others achieve their goals. It's about the connections you build, the support you offer, and the knowledge you share. My clients didn't care about my race times; they cared about the progress they made, the milestones they achieved, and the confidence they gained. I've found joy in helping others achieve their dreams and a sense of fulfillment in knowing that I'm making a difference.

I slowly started to pick up other clients through referrals and word of mouth. I still needed my day job, but I was getting closer to my dream of coaching full-time.

Just when I was actually building a business doing something I loved, the entire world turned upside down. At the beginning of 2020, the pandemic swept across the globe. Stay-at-home orders were issued, gyms and salons closed, races were canceled, schools sent kids home, and life as we knew it came to a halt.

Suddenly, I found myself without a job, at home with my preschooler. In Miami, the stay-at-home orders were strict: there were no more meetings at the beach for runs. Without any races to train for, being able to run or meet with my clients, or even leave the house for the gym or even my day job, that familiar darkness threatened to seep back into my life. This time, I refused to let it take hold.

I missed running so much, I wished I could go to the gym or head to the beach for a run, but that was not possible. Seeing how much I was missing this now huge part of my life, Donny, ever the supportive and encouraging partner, pulled out the credit card once again and bought me my very first treadmill, which was shipped and delivered right to our door. Now, as runners, we may refer to these as *dreadmills* because they're sometimes used only as a last resort for training. Sure, running in the same spot can be mind-numbingly boring. Of course, I'd much rather be running outside, especially when the beach is less than 4 miles away…but at some point, miles are miles. And at this point, I was desperate for a mental health run. I was so incredibly grateful to have my own *dreadmill* at home, in my garage. This allowed me to sneak in runs at Kylo's nap time or during the occasional screen time. *How convenient!* That one piece of equipment allowed me to train, keep my sanity during a very stressful time, and still be present for my little boy.

As much as I treasured the extra time with Kylo, I was not meant to be a stay-at-home mom. Even while the world was upside down, I still needed that driving force and purpose outside of the home. As a way to stay connected to the running community, I started a Facebook group and offered free running tips and advice in a supportive environment. This was a place for other moms and runners to come together. The group gave me something to do with my excess time and allowed me to continue to educate runners. In doing so, I gave myself a path to that fulfillment that I needed. But I missed getting to work closely with women one-on-one. That intimacy allowed me to give them personalized feedback and guidance on their journey.

After a few weeks of running the group, I decided to offer the members a free 20-minute coaching call so I could get to know them better and give them more individualized coaching. Angela was one of the very first women to take advantage of that free coaching call. We jumped on the phone and talked about everything from her recent divorce and raising her teenage son to her aspirations to start running and shed some weight.

I had no idea how to coach online, but I was confident I could help Angela reach her goals. She must have felt that way, too, because she asked about what coaching services I had to offer and signed up for my program right then and there, becoming my very first online client and the first official member of *Team Runderful.*

Angela's trust was the catalyst that propelled me forward. During the summer of 2020, an increasing number of women reached out to me, seeking support and guidance for their running or weight loss journeys. I embraced the opportunity and took the initiative to immerse myself in learning everything I could about running an online coaching business. I scoured YouTube for instructional videos and devoured podcast episodes. Every video I watched, or episode I listened to left me feeling more and more in control of my future.

Every evening, after putting my son to bed, I would stay up late into the night, trying to absorb all the information on building a successful coaching business that I could find. I learned how to create a website, create contracts, send invoices, accept payments, and manage the books for tax purposes. Each new skill felt like a step closer to my dream. If I encountered a problem, I put on my problem-solving hat and found a solution. With the invaluable help of Google University, my tenacity, and the unwavering faith of the founding members, *Something Runderful* was born. I even filed for an LLC.

I woke up some mornings wondering if everything that was happening around me was a dream. Growing up, I'd been told repeatedly by my dad that I needed to brush my hair at least 100 times a day in order to play up my looks and marry a rich husband. I'm ditzy by nature, but he joked constantly about how I wasn't a smart kid, and even called me hurtful nicknames. I knew he was joking, but still, I couldn't help but internalize the things he was saying.

For most of my life, I've felt like a disappointment. I had horrible grades, I'd been that angsty teenager who got lost in sex and drugs, and I'd gotten pregnant at 20 years old. *Who could be proud of a kid like that?* But now I had run a marathon, that same grueling 26.2 miles that my dad had completed all those years ago. I had a career that was gratifying. And at this point, I was so damn proud of the woman I had become. Regardless of the progress I had made, there was still part of me that continued to wonder if it was enough to make my parents proud. *Would I ever be good enough to make them proud?*

Building *Something Runderful* was not just about creating a business; it was about redefining my identity and proving to myself that I was more than my past mistakes. As the weeks turned into months, *Something Runderful* grew. The positive feedback from my clients fueled my passion and reassured me that I was on the right path. I formed meaningful connections with these women, sharing in their victories and supporting them through their struggles. The trust they placed in me was a constant source of motivation.

I mean, I was actually making a difference.

After I attempted to end my life, I wished desperately to find a purpose. *I mean, there had to be a reason I was still here, right?* Instead, I had to learn the hard way that I needed to create my own purpose. I believed that to bring purpose to my life, I needed to do something BIG, like change the entire world. But I have always felt small and insignificant, both physically and within the grand scheme of life. How could I, a 5-foot-tall, 20-something-year-old, have an impact on the world? It was then that I realized, I didn't need to change the entire world. I could have a big impact by just helping one person.

When I created *Something Runderful,* I committed to my deep belief in the ripple effect— that powerful, far-reaching magic that happens when you set out to inspire and uplift others.

For example, a mother who embraces running and achieves her goals sets a powerful example for her children. They see her dedication, her struggles, and her triumphs, they learn the values of discipline, resilience, and the importance of accomplishing goals. This impact doesn't stop with just her family. Her friends and coworkers who see her thriving might get inspired to lace up their own running shoes or start their own fitness journey. She may never know who will be inspired by her actions. Each person she touches creates another new ripple, spreading the wave of positive change even further. As a coach, it's honestly the best feeling to see my clients light up as they realize their own potential. Watching them inspire others and create their own ripples. Together we are changing the world, one woman at a time.

Something Runderful

Back in 7th grade, I was on the verge of failing Language Arts Class. As you know by now, I was not a good student and never took school seriously. Toward the end of the year, we had a final writing assignment. We had to write an essay about what our life would look like in the future: what we would do after college, what kind of career we would have, and what our lifestyle would be like. My teacher told me that if I wanted to get a passing grade for the class, I had to turn in this writing assignment. In true young Ally fashion, I just procrastinated until the very last minute. And by last minute, I mean I was brushing my teeth and getting ready for bed when suddenly I remembered that the paper was due the next day. I went to my mom, panicking. *"Mom! My paper is due tomorrow, I don't want to fail English class and have to redo it next year. Please help me!"*

To my relief, my mom said, *"Okay, I'll do the paper for you."* Now, this wasn't the first time my mom had saved my butt by doing a late-night project for me. She knew at this point that I couldn't care less about school. She might not have held me accountable to doing my nightly homework or stayed on top of what my grades were, but she would always swoop in to help me when I needed it. My mom was likely enabling me, but I was so grateful she was willing to save me one more time.

"Go to sleep, I'll start working on your paper, and I'll have it done by tomorrow morning."

In the morning, I awoke to find my mom still at the computer typing. I asked to read the paper, and my mom brushed me away, *"No, no, it's not done yet. But I promise to finish the paper and drop it off to you at school."* Okay, that's fine, my Language Arts Class wasn't until later in the afternoon. I sat in school, class after class, getting more nervous as time ticked by. As I headed to lunch my mom still hadn't brought me my paper and I really started to panic. *What if she forgot? What if she wasn't bringing it just to teach me a lesson?* I know now just as well as I knew then that I am the guilty one here, but I was terrified. I was not ready to go to class and admit to my teacher that I didn't do the assignment and deal with the consequence of ultimately failing 7th grade English.

Just as the bell rang for us to head to Language Arts Class, I heard my name on the overhead speaker. I was being called to the office. With a huge sigh of relief, I started sprinting towards the front of the school. I picked up my paper from the office with just enough time to rush to class before the final tardy bell. I made it to my desk just in time. *Now, I finally have the chance to read the paper my mom wrote on my behalf.* I read the title; *I am a Gardener. What the heck?* Out of all the things my mom could have written about, she wrote about me becoming a GARDENER?!? I didn't even like getting my hands dirty, let alone having the patience to try growing anything. I was absolutely baffled, but before I could read further, my teacher called on me. *"Ally, why don't you come up to the front of the class and read us your paper."*

If I wasn't already sweating from my sprint to class, I was sure sweating now. I hadn't even gotten to read this essay to myself and now I had to read it aloud for all of my peers.

I wish I still had a copy of this paper many years later, but I do remember most of it. Here's a basic summary:

The paper started off with me as a young adult with a passion and talent for photography. I went around taking pictures of people and making them feel beautiful. One day, I happened to be walking in the park with my camera, when I came across an attractive guy throwing a frisbee with his dog. Inspired, I started to capture candid pictures of this man playing with his dog. I ended up showing him the images, and I guess we fell in love and got married. The rest of the paper ended up being whimsical, dramatic and full of life lessons. Where does the gardening aspect come in? Well, it was woven into the paper as a metaphor for the beautiful life I'd cultivated and nurtured. Because I was the one responsible for my life, the one tending to my own growth, I was the gardener of my own life. The essay concluded with this final sentence. I am a moody, compassionate, creative, overall kind of a dumb teenager on the verge of something wonderful.

Walking back to my desk, I was beyond embarrassed. My mom must have just been laughing her butt off when she wrote this paper. Given how poorly I had done on my other work for this class and my completely different writing style, there was no way in hell the teacher was going to believe that I wrote this essay. The other kids in my class wrote very straightforward papers about going to college, getting a job in a prestigious career, or traveling the world. And I got to read this whimsical metaphorical drama. I couldn't help but laugh.

But that last line kept repeating in my mind.

I am a moody, compassionate, creative, overall kind of a dumb teenager on the verge of something wonderful.

It's like my mom was having a little dig at me. She knew I was an irresponsible kid who had made mistakes, but I still had the potential to create a beautiful life.

I ended up passing my class, but I didn't exactly learn my lesson because I still needed my mom to help me with a couple more future projects. My grades didn't improve, and I may have missed out on the valuable lesson of either putting in the work myself or failing. Yet, I still carried that last sentence with me.

I *was* a kind of dumb teenager on the verge of something wonderful.

When I had my son, I was a kind of dumb new mom on the verge of something wonderful.

And when I started running, *I was a kind of a dumb redhead on the verge of Something RUNDERFUL.*

In life, there are moments when we feel on the verge of something transformative, something wonderful, teetering on the brink of discovering our true potential. Regardless of the potential we see before us, we won't obtain it until we take responsibility for ourselves and do the work.

Something Runderful wasn't just a catchy phrase I came up with on a whim; It symbolizes how every mistake I've made, every stumble I've taken along the way, has contributed to my evolution and shaped the person I am today. When I was coming up with the name of my brand, my business, and my values as a coach, I kept coming back to *Something Runderful*.

It reminds me—and now my clients—that our paths are filled with opportunities to learn, grow, and shine, no matter how many times we fall.

My clients are the living embodiment of *Something Runderful*. When I tell them they are *something runderful*, it's not because they've achieved perfection or have it all figured out. It's because they've dared to embark on their individual journeys, willing to embrace the ups and downs.

Something Runderful serves as a constant reminder to my clients to look back on how far they've come. It encourages them to celebrate their progress, no matter how small, and to keep pushing toward the goals and dreams they have yet to accomplish. It's a call to embrace the journey, with all its imperfections and challenges, and to recognize the beauty in their mistakes and past *dumb* decisions.

After Angela and I had been working together for just over a year, she brought up the idea of coming to Florida to participate in a South Florida Half Marathon so that we could run it together. At this point, she'd accomplished incredible milestones: running her first 5k, 10k, and half marathon. And even though we had been training together virtually, we had never met in person. Donny was sitting next to me when I told him that I was excited about potentially running a race in person with Angela. He immediately asked for my phone. *(One amazing thing about my husband is that he's not just my cheerleader but yours too.)* He dialed up Angela. His voice filled with enthusiasm as he said, *"If you're coming all the way to South Florida, you're not just doing a half marathon. You better be running the full marathon."* There was a moment of stunned silence, followed by Angela's nervous laughter. After swearing she would never run a marathon, she agreed right then and there to tackle the Miami Marathon with me.

Since Angela was driving down to run the race, we decided to extend the invitation to some of the other members of our virtual running community. Three other incredible women joined us: Mackenzie and Kelly, both agreeing to run their first marathons, and another woman opting for the half marathon.

For me, running the Miami Marathon again was deeply personal. It was the race that had marked the beginning of my own journey, a place where I had once struggled and persevered. Now, I was coming full circle, ready to share this transformative experience with the very women I had been coaching.

The race was at the end of January, which is a beautiful time of year in Miami. While there's always humidity, the actual temperatures are amazing. Lows are in the 60s, with highs in the 70s. Our team was coming from various parts of the country, many escaping the chill of winter for the warmth and sunshine of South Florida.

Getting to meet a few of my clients in person was an absolute dream come true.

I was nervous though. My online persona is outgoing, bubbly, and highly energetic. However, in person, I can sometimes be awkward, standoffish, and quiet. In social situations, a nasty voice in the back of my head starts to speak up, telling me that girls are mean and gossipy and will do something to emotionally hurt me. But everything changed when I decided to create my own community, carefully cultivating my tribe with love and intention.

The first in-person meeting with my long-distance clients was absolutely magic. Not only was I at ease, but I witnessed their friendships blossom, and I saw how easily everyone got along. These strangers from different walks of life and areas of the country became such fast friends and support systems for each other. They came together to do something that scared and excites them. In the few days we all spent together in Florida, they helped rewrite the story I had told myself for all those years about girls and women being mean. I realized how beautiful that connection can really be when women choose to empower each other.

The morning of the race, I woke up early, bright-eyed and excited, sipping on a cup of coffee while my clients were still rubbing the sleep from their eyes.

I was buzzing with excitement, but we could all feel the nerves in the room. As thrilled as I was for them and for the experience they were going to have, I was also trying to be mindful of the nerves I knew they were dealing with. I could, and still can, clearly remember the feelings before my first race, the Miami Marathon.

Before the race, I gathered the team and reminded them to run their own races. As a coach, my role was to support them, I was committed to running alongside whoever needed me the most to ensure no one was left behind. Based on their training, it looked like Kelly would lead the way, with Angela not far behind, and Mackenzie, who had battled COVID during training, would bring up the rear.

As the race began, I stayed close to Mackenzie, while Angela and Kelly surged ahead. Around mile 7, we were surprised to catch back up with Kelly as we ran through the iconic streets of South Beach. "*What's going on, Kelly? How are you feeling?*" I asked.

Kelly, visibly struggling, admitted that the Miami heat was getting to her. She had spent all winter training in the frigid, snowy conditions of her hometown. Battling frostbite and hypothermia on her long runs, not heat exhaustion and dehydration. Her body wasn't reacting well to the warmth and humidity of Florida, and she had to take frequent breaks to stretch and walk. Mackenzie and I stuck by her side, offering words of encouragement and support.

After a few miles of the three of us sticking together, I had to break up the trio. I turned to Mackenzie. "*You have to go ahead. You have to go run your own race.*" Mackenzie was hesitant to run ahead, leaving us behind, but I reminded her again that this was *her* race. With this encouragement, she finally took off. I can't tell you how proud I felt at that moment. I was like a mama bird gently kicking her chick out of the nest. Watching my client, Mackenzie, as she ran up ahead, crossing over the bridge that heads into downtown, will be a memory I cherish forever.

At Mile 11, Kelly was really struggling. So, I told her, "*Kelly, if you just get to mile 13, you can stop at the half-marathon finish.*" I don't know if there was a tone in my voice, or if Kelly just knew me well enough to know that no matter what I was saying, I was not going to let her switch to running only the half marathon, unless it became unsafe for her to continue. But my offer gave her a bite-sized goal that got her through some of the hardest miles.

Luckily, as we ran through the city, skyscrapers shadowed the roads, finally providing some much-needed relief from the harsh Miami sun.

As we approached the barricades that divided those running the half marathon from those running the full marathon, I remembered the feelings I'd had during my first marathon; wanting desperately to quit and choosing to keep going. I kept silent, half a step behind Kelly, and I watched with pride as she made that same choice. Kelly veered towards the marathon route, determined to continue with the full marathon as she'd planned. As we ran on, I was reminded that in these races quitting is always an option, but there's so much more to be gained when we stick to the goals we set for ourselves, in experience, pride, and bragging rights. It was special watching Kelly make that decision for herself.

As the race went on, the day only continued to heat up.

I texted my husband that we needed ice. He hopped on his motorcycle and went off on an emergency mission. He was quick and met us along the course a few miles later. We took that ice and stuffed it into Kelly's sports bra to cool the core of her body down. (*Bloody toenails and boob ice - running a marathon is super sexy, isn't it?*) At aid stations, I was dumping Dixie cups full of water on the back of her neck. Our efforts were working to keep Kelly cooled down enough to keep her moving forward.

Between the excess heat, sweat, and water we were drenching Kelly with though, a new problem became apparent at mile 18. The abundance of moisture created hot spots and gigantic blisters on the bottom of her feet. This development caused her significant discomfort and hindered her gait until her running turned into more of a painful limping.

Kelly looked at me and frantically asked, *"Ally, am I going faster when I am running or walking?"*

As a momma of two kids, Kelly started comparing the race to giving birth, saying that running this marathon was harder and longer than any labor she had endured. Yet she kept pushing through the pain, step by agonizing step, never quitting, never surrendering. It was like I was watching Kelly struggling down her own green hallway.

I was so proud of Kelly and all that she was accomplishing for herself. At the same time, I kept flashing back to my own struggles. The times when I could feel that familiar darkness creeping in, threatening to stop me in my tracks, when I could barely walk without the support of a walker. Until I ran with Kelly, I had never understood what people mean when they say things have come full circle. In being with Kelly while she trudged on, getting to cheer her on and support her through the process, I was becoming the person I had wanted and needed through my hardest struggles, during my first marathon... I was becoming the type of person I had needed earlier in my life.

When we were about 100 yards from the finish line, I looked at Kelly, my vision blurred by the tears welling in my eyes. "*You've got this. I'll see you at the finish line,*" I said. I sprinted ahead, throwing out my arms and flying across the finish line. As soon as I'd crossed, I snagged not one medal but two. As Kelly officially became a Marathon Finisher, I placed the medal around her neck. We embraced each other, exhausted, drained, and ugly crying from all of the bottled-up emotions from the day. It was such an honor that I'd been able to play even a small role in this amazing woman achieving such a monumental goal.

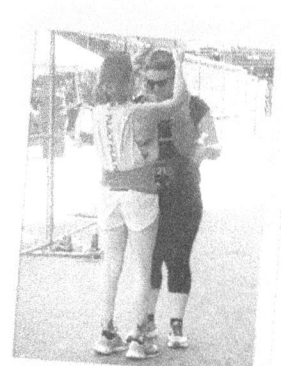

Kelly's first marathon medal

In all the races I've run on my own, the races in which I've paced clients, and the clients I've coached, I have never experienced anything quite like this. The struggle, the fight, and the sheer determination Kelly displayed were awe-inspiring and unbelievably beautiful to witness firsthand. Maybe my mom was right: we are the "gardeners" of our own lives.

Kelly's journey through the Miami Marathon epitomizes the essence of *Something Runderful.* Faced with heat, painful blisters, and the temptation to quit, she chose perseverance over comfort. We are all on the brink of something wonderful, and through our challenges, we become *something runderful.*

Ally Robinson

Where Angels Land

Every year around the Fourth of July, my parents would load us kids into the car, stuffing the trunk with camping gear, snacks, and hiking boots, and drive up to Zion National Park in Utah. This was my absolute favorite trip of the year (even more than Disneyland). Some years, we even went with family friends who had kids around our age. I always looked forward to a week of fun hiking, exploring, and seeing the most beautiful scenery ever. My heart would race when we approached the 1-mile tunnel that we had to go through to get to the National Park. My brother and I would try to hold our breath for the whole tunnel but always ended up gasping for air before we reached the other side.

The days were filled with endless exploration. We'd hike trails that wound through narrow canyons, past waterfalls, and over rocky terrain. My favorite part was always The Narrows. This is a hike that requires us to walk in the Virgin River, where sometimes we'd even have to swim upstream between the red rocks of Zion. When we got tired from hiking, we could stop and play in the cool, refreshing water. We'd splash around and jump off rocks into the water below and then relax on the riverbank, munching on jerky and drinking Tang.

There was one trail that was off-limits to us kids though, Angel's Landing. It's a massive rock formation that seemed to touch the sky, and the legend was that only angels could land on it. The hike to the top was notoriously dangerous, with steep inclines and deadly drop-offs. People have even lost their lives attempting to ascend it. The adults would take turns going on this hike while the others stayed back with us kids, but I always dreamed of standing where the angels stood and looking out over the breathtaking landscape.

When I turned 9, my parents finally agreed to let me attempt the Angel's Landing trail. I was ecstatic, a mix of excitement and nerves buzzing inside me. The years of anticipation and the thrill of the danger drew me in. I was determined to prove myself. For a 9-year-old, I was pretty athletic, thanks to years of ballet, but this hike was unlike anything I had ever experienced.

The trail started off easy enough, winding through shaded trees and alongside the river. But soon, it started to ascend. The path became steeper, and the drop-offs more sheer. My legs burned with effort, and my heart pounded in my chest. I was both terrified and exhilarated. There was a section of the trail known as Walter's Wiggles, a series of 21 tight switchbacks that seemed to go on forever. Each step felt like a victory, bringing me closer to my goal.

Then came the final stretch——the infamous narrow ridge. There was barely enough room to put one foot in front of the other, and the only thing to hold onto was a chain drilled into the rock. The chain was my lifeline, the only thing standing between me and a sheer drop to the canyon floor below. I gripped it so tightly that my knuckles turned white. I wasn't scared of heights, but this was a whole new level of insanity.

"Don't look down," my mom said, but then she noticed that my eyes were squeezed completely closed. *"Ally! You have to open your eyes!"*

I forced myself to look. The world seemed to spin around me, but I took a deep breath and focused on the trail ahead. At one point, I was so scared to stand that I dropped to my hands and knees, crawling along the narrow path. My heart was hammering, but I didn't give up.

Finally, we reached the top. The view was even more incredible than I had imagined. The canyon spread out below, a sea of red rock. I had done it! I had braved Angel's Landing, and it was everything I had dreamed it would be.

This was the last summer of our annual Zion trip. For years I dreamed about going back and conquering the scary trail again, but life happened. We moved to that moldy house, my sister was sick, and the days of hiking and swimming in the river were nothing but distant memories.

Before my family moved to Florida, they decided to take one last trip to Zion National Park. I felt the same thrill I had nearly ten years prior. Zion's magic never faded, no matter how many times we visited.

While I looked forward to all the nostalgic activities, we would be filling our days with, the thing I was most looking forward to was going back to Angel's Landing. This time, I knew what to expect as we approached the imposing red rock. The first glimpse of those towering cliffs brought back a flood of memories. I remembered the adrenaline that coursed through my veins the first time I stood at the base, staring up at what seemed like an insurmountable challenge.

Even though it was years later, I felt like I remembered every twist and turn of the trail, every steep incline and narrow ledge. The knowledge of the path ahead gave me a sense of comfort. The sections that had once filled me with dread now felt like an old friend, familiar and manageable. The hike wasn't as daunting as I had remembered. Maybe it was because I was older, or it could have been because I knew what to expect this time. Either way, I felt a calm confidence as we made our way up the trail.

As we hiked, I thought back to that moment years ago when I had been too scared to stand, crawling on my hands and knees, my heart pounding in my chest. The narrow ridge, with its dizzying drop-offs and only the chain to hold onto, had seemed impossible back then. But now, in that same spot, I stood tall and unafraid. I even posed for a picture to capture my transformation.

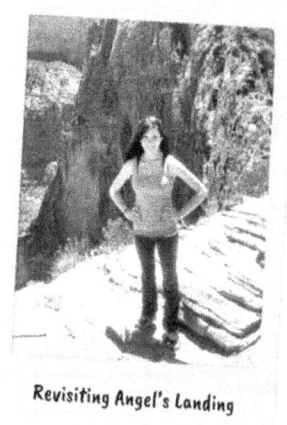

Revisiting Angel's Landing

As a coach, I often reflect on that hike when talking to my athletes. I laugh when people tell me they are only going to run one marathon—*one and done,* they say. For some, that might be true, but I know a different truth. The first time is always the hardest, filled with uncertainties and so many unknowns. It's an exhilarating experience, but it can also be overwhelming. *Is it even possible to fully appreciate the experience when it's so new and daunting?*

I've seen plenty of athletes start with the intention of running just one marathon, only to come back months or even years later, excited and determined to do another. These accidental repeat marathoners tell me how much they learned from their first experience and that they'd like to try again. Some want to go faster, others commit to preparing better, and almost all of them want to enjoy the experience more the second time around. The first marathon teaches you a lot about yourself, about pushing through limits, and about the sheer joy of crossing the finish line.

There is no comparing future experiences to the first time. If I had given up on running after my first miserable experience, I would have missed out on so many amazing adventures. Running has taken me to incredible places, introduced me to inspiring people, and taught me lessons that go beyond the sport itself.

The hike up Angel's Landing was more than just a physical challenge; it was an analogy for all the obstacles and fears we face in life. Each time we push through, we become stronger and more confident. When we look back, we see how far we've come and how those first steps, no matter how shaky, were the beginning of something extraordinary.

Ally Robinson

AROO!

After several years of being a running coach, I had officially made running my entire life. Turning a hobby into a career isn't always appropriate. In fact, many people have shared that it slowly destroys the love they feel for their hobby. Fortunately, I still loved running, but my desire to train and run my own races was dwindling as I dedicated focus to helping my clients cross their finish lines and achieve their new PRs.

A friend of mine mentioned that she was training for an upcoming Spartan Race. At the time, I had never even heard of Spartan races or any other kind of OCR *(obstacle course race)* before. She gushed about how fun it was. *"It's like a race but with obstacles, like climbing over 6-foot walls, crawling under barbed wire through mud, and throwing a spear."*

That was exactly what I was looking for to bring some spice and excitement back to my own running practice!

Without much knowledge or preparation, I dove headfirst into the Spartan world, signing up for the next available race near my home. Little did I know that Spartan races had different competition levels, and I naively entered the Age Group category. I was totally unaware that it was a competitive wave demanding penalties of 30 burpees for each failed obstacle. For those who aren't familiar with the Spartan world, this means that for every obstacle I failed to overcome, I would have to stop what I was doing and complete 30 burpees before continuing with the race. While I was no stranger to strength training, I certainly had never done 30 burpees in a row. Let alone multiple sets of 30 burpees during a single race. When I showed up to the race and actually learned the rules, I was absolutely flabbergasted. As a seasoned road runner, I'd come into my first Spartan race thinking it would just be another cool race to conquer, another medal for my growing collection at home. *It's a 5k, how hard could that be?* Instead, it humbled me completely.

When I got to the event, it was a huge festival. Just to get to the start line, you have to get over a 4ft wall. I *tried*, unsuccessfully, to climb over it as gracefully as I saw the other Spartans do it. In the starting line corral, runners introduced themselves to each other, high fiving, and chatting amongst themselves like old friends. *This was unlike any other starting line vibe I had ever experienced.* When it was time to start the race, there was a man with a speakerphone shouting, *"Who are you?"* To which the crowd of runners responded, *"I Am A*

Spartan!" This chanting went on a few times, with the excitement culminating in a resounding *AROO, AROO, AROO* before the voice shouted - *"GO!"* The only way I can think of to describe it is that the spirit of camaraderie in Spartan races touched my soul. No matter what happened over the next few miles, I knew that I'd found my tribe.

The rest of the race day was a brutal awakening. Spartan obstacles required so much more than just strength. Many of these obstacles required technique and strategy, which I definitely didn't have at the time. I failed so many obstacles in that first race. Which means I also did more burpees than I ever could have imagined. Thankfully, what I lacked in upper body strength and skill, I made up for in running speed, but geez, by the end, I was exhausted. I hardly had enough energy to lift my arms above my head and jump over the fire for the iconic Spartan finish. That last obstacle is well known in the OCR world, but I didn't even know that fire, yes, with real flames, would be a part of any obstacle. Talk about an experience. When I finally crossed the finish line of that first Spartan race, I'd managed to place 2nd in my age group.

At the time, I was so mentally and emotionally defeated from failing so many obstacles that I didn't even bother to check my placement after the race. I didn't even know that I'd podiumed on my very first Spartan race until I got home later that night. *For those of you who aren't crazy runners like I am, it's a HUGE deal to earn a spot on the podium, and to not stick around for that moment of glory and recognition is basically a huge party foul.*

When I was back at home, icing my muscles, and licking my wounds, I started reflecting on the idea of the penalties throughout the race. Sure, we can all agree that burpees suck, and so does failing obstacles, but I realized that just because you don't master something on the first attempt, it doesn't mean that you've lost, that the race is over, or that you should quit. Hell no, you take your penalty, do the 30-burpees, and keep going. This isn't just a great lesson when it comes to running; it pertains to every aspect of life. And while those penalties do suck at the time, they also help make us stronger and more resilient in our next race, or in our next chapter of life.

That first race started what I now think of as a Spartan itch… I wanted to get better at those obstacles, especially the ones that had seriously kicked my ass.

Determined to excel, I joined an OCR gym. When walking in the front door, it was as though I had entered a little baby monkey's dream house. It was filled from floor to ceiling, wall to wall, with climbing equipment and obstacles to practice on. The entire space smelled like sweat, determination, and future Spartan medals. Many of the things I saw were actually the obstacles that had given me the most trouble during that first race.

The gym was owned by a man who regularly did burpees for breakfast and exuded the spirit of Spartan racing. *Literally. On Instagram, he went live and did 100 burpees every single morning, it's crazy.* During the classes at the gym, he'd demonstrate how to tackle each obstacle. He made it look absolutely effortless.

I knew right away that he was the coach for me.

In the world of Spartan races, there are different distances. Each distance has a different name, which makes it much easier for us racers to know and communicate what we're training for with our fellow crazy OCR runners. The breakdown is:

Spartan Sprint - 5k - 20 obstacles

Spartan Super - 10k - 25 obstacles

Spartan Beast - Half Marathon - 30 obstacles

And then *(insert gladiator-like theme music here)*

The Spartan ULTRA - 30+ miles - 60 obstacles

As an athlete, I am on this never-ending journey to push my limits. I decided that after conquering the sprint, super, and beast, it just made sense for me to take on the Spartan Ultra. My mileage was already there, as I had recently finished running several marathons on back-to-back weekends. *(Yes, I'd become that girl who ate, drank, slept, and breathed running.)* But running long distances in a road race is way different than running long distances on trails. It's even more challenging during a Spartan race where the path takes you over treacherous rocks, through knee-high grass, sludging through swamps, wading through rivers or lakes, and clambering up insane structures meant to keep even the most determined person out. No number of marathons would ever prepare me for the 9+ hours of hell that my first Spartan Ultra put me through.

This was the first race since my first marathon where I was nervous, like knee-shaking, stomachache, maybe I should just stay home in bed, nervous. That's when I first realized the big difference between self-confidence and self-assurance. My self-confidence was shaken. *What if I failed? What if it was just too hard?* But my self-assurance was strong, *I am trained for this. I am as prepared as possible. I've got this!*

In past Spartan races, I'd relied on my nature as a runner to outrun the competition, but in a 30+ mile race, starting out too fast is actually a really bad idea. My goal for this race was to place first for my age group, so I needed to make smart decisions. Somewhere around mile 6, I had this woman right on my tail... so I kept pushing faster, trying to lose her. Each time I increased my pace, she matched me. *Ugh. I couldn't shake her.* Finally, I yelled over my shoulder. *How old are you?* She shouted back and ended up being quite a few years older than me, placing her in a different age group. Ah, wonderful! While we were still racing, she wasn't my direct competitor. This meant that running together wouldn't negatively impact either of us getting first place in our age group. We both slowed our pace once we knew that we could be friends throughout the race. We talked about our kids, our careers, and the crazy thought process that had led to us signing up for an Ultra Obstacle Course Race. I was grateful to have her company. It's against the rules in Spartan races to wear headphones, so there are hours and hours where it's just you and your own thoughts as boredom and fatigue set in. Getting to spend some quality time with another athlete is a blessing.

There was a point in the race where we split up and continued at our own pace. This was fine until I realized that I'd been running, in the forest, by myself for quite a ways. I started to feel completely alone, and the only reason I knew I was still on the right track were the markers that had been put out by the race organizers. Finally, the silence got to me, and I sang out, *"Ole, Ole, Ole, Ole" (which is apparently some soccer anthem, but it was the first thing that came to mind).* A few seconds later, in the distance, I heard the soft echo of a male's voice bouncing off the canyon walls, *"Ole, Ole."* Whew. I knew I wasn't alone, and that there was someone not too far ahead of me.

At the 15-ish mile mark, it started to rain. This meant the obstacles were wet, which made things like rope climbs and monkey bars even more difficult. Even though this North Carolina Ultra Race was advertised as being flat... it definitely wasn't. Whoever said the course was flat needs to look up the definition in the dictionary because there were parts of this race that were anything but flat. Steep uphill climbs were followed by tough descents. Those downhills turned into mudslides after a few minutes of rain. All of us Spartans had to go slowly and carefully on the slippery declines to avoid falling, but in the true spirit of working smarter, not harder, I sat my butt down on the slippery mud and slid my way down the hills. Sure, I had literally no control over where I landed and nearly died a few times from crashing into a tree or two on my way down. Luckily though, my pants didn't rip and expose my rear end for the remainder of the race, and I got to the bottom twice as fast as anyone else.

All throughout training, I had anticipated and prepared for how hard this race would be, so for the first 2/3rds of the race, even though I was filthy, exhausted, and still had hours ahead of me, I was having so much fun. I was fortunate to find a few different groups of people along the way, to chat with. But eventually, the miles started to catch up with me and my calves cramped up so badly that it was painful to run. Around mile 29, I started thinking about the green hallway again. It's crazy how fast I could go from feeling great to barely being able to lift my arms. How much my back hurt. Each time I jumped down from an obstacle it felt like every vertebra in my back was compressing into the next. On one of the rope obstacles, the rope dug against my cuticle, ripping my skin away and covering my hand with blood for the rest of the race.

During the race, I was so tough, doing what Spartans do, holding it all together, gritting my teeth, and pushing through the pain and exhaustion. But the moment I saw my husband, I couldn't hold it back anymore, and the waterworks started. He was my safe person, and seeing him there, in the rain, cheering me on allowed me to let all of my emotions flow. That's the thing, in a tough race, and really in life, we don't have to suppress those negative emotions. Letting them flow can be such a healing release. Once I stopped focusing so much of my energy on keeping it together, I was able to move past the negative feelings, move on, and keep pushing forward.

At mile 30, there was an obstacle that stopped me in my tracks. It was a smooth inclined wall where I had to run up and grab onto a rope before pulling myself the rest of the way up and over the wall. Let me tell you, they don't call it a slip-wall for no reason. And after all of the rain and mud, there was nothing but slip for both me and the wall. Now, I want to remind you here that I am a tiny person, like, seriously short. And this wall was massive, the rope hanging impossibly high.

On my first attempt up the wall, I ran up, my shoes lost traction, and I landed hard on my belly, sliding back down the wall and into the mud. After 30 miles, and hours and hours of running, crawling, jumping, and climbing, I was out of steam. I stood back up, took a deep breath, gritted my teeth, and ran as fast as I could using any momentum I could gain, to lift myself off the ground and hopefully grab onto the rope. Again, I slid back down to the ground. I didn't know how I was going to do this. Every attempt took more and more energy out of me, and while I was determined to conquer this obstacle, I wasn't sure if I'd be able to actually do it. Of course, this wall was one of the few obstacles in the Spartan Ultra race that you can't burpee your way out of. Either you get up and over the wall, or you DNF *(Did Not Finish)* and there was absolutely no way in hell that I was about to drop out in the last few miles of the race. So again, I ran towards the wall. My fingertips brushed the rope, and I slid back down

scan here to see the
video clip

like I had so many times already. I screamed in anger and frustration. But I choose to give it another go. Again. I slipped... Again, this time my fingers touched the rope, but the mud made it just as slick as the wall, and again, it slipped through my fingers. Tears welled up in my eyes, and I was, for the first time, afraid that I wasn't going to be able to finish the race. I knew that my body wasn't going to put up with this much longer.

I only had enough energy to try one more time. And, on my 7th attempt, I felt my hand contact with the rope like a magnet. The world around me moved in slow motion. I gripped the rope and pulled my body up and over the wall. I did it.

Leaping over the iconic Spartan Fire, I finished the race in 9hr and 40-some minutes, earning 1st place in my age group.

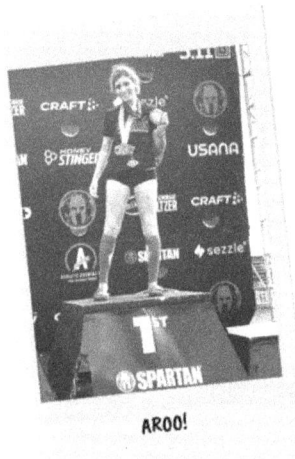

AROO!

This is the race that prompted David Covington to message me one last time in regard to sharing my story in his film. Because of that, when I think back to all my races, it's this one that always stands out as a monumental moment in my life. Not only did this race start the ball rolling with me sharing my story in David's film, and ultimately writing this book, but placing first in my age group qualified me for the Spartan Ultra World Championships. This was a grueling 24-hour Spartan race and was taking place in the mountains of Lake Tahoe later that year.

I only had about four months to train for the World Championship, and it became part of my personality. I worked with my clients, took care of my son, and trained for hours and hours every single day.

My entire life became about putting my mind and body through all sorts of hell. I even did a 24-hour running challenge: one mile every hour for 24 hours. *1/10 - 0 out of 5 stars— do not recommend it!!!* As absolutely horrible as the experience was, it made me appreciate what I could accomplish in an utterly sleep-deprived state. In order to get my body acclimated to the freezing cold temperatures that awaited me in Tahoe, I also did ocean plunges and ice baths. Seriously, I would rather run through the depths of hell than have to sit in another ice bath for 2 minutes.

Hypothermia in July

While training for the Spartan Ultra World Championship, I ran my first 50-mile race. Even registering for the race is a bit of a funny story because I never really had any intentions of running a 50-mile race. It all started because of a t-shirt. After my winning performance at the Ultra Spartan, my client Mackenzie *(remember, my amazing clients that ran ahead of us in the Miami Marathon?)* sent me a t-shirt that said, *"Look at me running ultra-marathons and shit."* I absolutely loved the shirt and wore it all the time with pride. But then my husband commented. *"You didn't run an ultra-marathon, you ran an ultra-Spartan, it's different."* For someone who doesn't even run, I found his comment humorous but also more than slightly infuriating. *Anything over 26.2 miles is an ultra. An ultra is an ultra and an incredible feat. But whatever, I see your point. I guess I need to sign up for an ultra-marathon.* The next local ultra marathon race was 50-miler in July, in Florida. This race ended up being a great learning experience that physically and mentally prepared me for whatever races I might want to tackle in the future. *So, thanks, Mackenzie.*

I dedicated myself to an intense training regimen, running 40-60 miles weekly to prepare for this ultra marathon. I tried to run at the hottest parts of the day to acclimate to the heat. Regardless of how I trained, I knew there was really no way around it; This race was going to be brutally hot.

I found immense comfort in knowing my best friend, Dawn, was going to be there to crew for me. Dawn wasn't just any friend; she had been by my side for years. Even though she's ten years older than I am, we have a deep sisterly bond. We were both pregnant at the same time with our first children and connected over the trials and tribulations of pregnancy and motherhood. We also share a crazy love for running.

Dawn has a long history as a runner, starting with cross country training at the local high school when she was just in 7th grade. When she was officially able to run for the high school team, they made it to the state championship every year. She went on to run her freshman year in college before deciding to keep running as a hobby rather than a job. Dawn even ran throughout her pregnancy, finishing second place for her age group at almost 8 months pregnant. I always enjoyed hearing her stories about competing in 5k and 10k races. When I first started running, I would have loved to run with Dawn, but I was so embarrassed by my slow pace. I didn't even tell her I was running. There was no way I could keep up with how fast she was. But I still tried. I often tried to match her running pace on my own, pushing myself to keep up, but could only sustain it for a minute or two before reaching my limit. Of course, trying to push harder and run faster than my body could handle was ultimately what led to my injuries. This constant comparison led to frustration and feelings of inadequacy. I wanted so badly to be on her level that I ignored my own body's signals, which only set me back further.

It wasn't until after my first marathon, that horrible yet exhilarating experience, that I decided to stop comparing myself to others and to start focusing on my own progress. I hired a coach, and she created a personalized training plan tailored to my current fitness level. As I progressed and got better with my running, while concentrating only on a better version of myself and beating my own PRs, something unexpected happened. I was getting faster and improving by leaps and bounds. I actually started to be able to keep up with Dawn's pace and eventually surpassed her 5k race pace. It wasn't about beating Dawn, though. We still hadn't even run together! It was about the valuable lesson I learned; to stay in my own lane.

It taught me that progress is deeply personal and that my value as a runner and as a person wasn't defined by how I stacked up to others. If I had continued to measure my ability as a runner based on just trying to keep up with Dawn, I would have eventually given up, burned out, or been injured to a point of no return.

Before I ran my first marathon, Dawn ended up moving 6 hours away. Despite the distance, throughout all my running years, she has been there every step of the way, celebrating my victories and comforting me during setbacks. Our bond grew stronger as we supported each other's journeys from afar.

Dawn had a goal of PR'ing a 15k race which is held every year in Jacksonville, Florida. I'd heard her talking about this race before, mentioning how at some point in the race, spectators actually throw donut holes at the runners. And I love donuts, so I made the decision that I was going to run this iconic race, and it was going to be the very first time I actually ran with my best friend. During the race, I paced Dawn, as her friend and coach, and she ultimately beat her goal time by nearly 3 minutes. I even got to eat a donut mid run after Dawn caught it midair and handed to me. I had so much fun getting to run this race with her.

When I needed to start thinking about who I wanted to crew me for my 50-miler, I knew Dawn would be the ideal crew member: she's my best friend, a fellow runner, and an ICU nurse with a background in athletic training. She was the best person to have supported me during this race.

The morning of my 50-mile race, I stuck to my tried-and-true pre-race meal: instant mashed potatoes. Simple, packed with carbs and sodium, and easy to prepare in our hotel room. Although, I couldn't sleep. I can never sleep very well before a race. I was up long before my alarm went off. This gave me plenty of time to eat, get ready, and nervously pace the hotel room while Dawn slept in until 5 a.m.

As I stood at the starting line, I couldn't help but notice how much younger I was than all of the other participants. I was the third youngest out of the hundreds of runners, a fact that filled me with a mixture of pride and apprehension. *What the heck was I getting myself into?* Even though it was 6 a.m. the Florida heat was already making its presence known.

The first few miles were surreal as we ran along the beach, watching the sunrise. As a Miami runner, I often train along the ocean, but this experience was magical. The beach we were running on is known for being a sea turtle nesting ground. Mamma turtles come up onto the beach at night and lay their eggs before returning back to sea before dawn. As we were running along the ocean, we could actually see the imprints in the sand that the momma sea turtles had left the night before: her smooth belly, and the indents of her flippers. One philosophy I have always carried with me is to, *"Never run so fast that you forget to watch the sunrise."* This life lesson helped keep my ego in check through the first few miles of the race. It reminded me to slow down, take in the beautiful sunrise, and just enjoy the moments. The problem with that very early on I found myself, once again, in no man's land.

I wasn't upfront with the speed goats, but I wasn't back with the slower crowd either. I thrive off the energy of running with people. Even if we aren't talking, just having someone to pace with and run next to can make a huge difference in the enjoyment of, and ultimately my performance in a race. I knew I didn't want to end up all alone, so I considered whether I wanted to speed up or slow down to find a companion but decided ultimately, to stick to my own pace. This was my race, at my pace.

Running your own race is sound advice, but this was particularly true in these first few miles. I started to find myself in a very uncomfortable situation way too early on in this race. I am no stranger to sandy runs, but the challenge for me was that this beach had a steep angle sloping towards the ocean. Running in the same direction for a long period of time on the uneven surface quickly started to wreak havoc on my hips, especially my hip flexor. To avoid thinking about the loneliness and the uncomfortable running situation, I started looking around for things to help occupy my brain. Looking down, I started to notice these big beautiful, intact white shells. So, every mile, I would bend down and scoop up a shell, stashing it into my running vest as a memento of the journey. I'm sure Dawn was more than a little surprised and amused when she was cleaning out my vest, finding it filled with seashells. I knew she noticed them because they were gone the next time I traded in for that vest.

Eventually, we left the beach for the pavement, a welcome change despite the harder impact on my joints. I knew I would soon see Dawn, my one-woman crew, waiting to support me. We had planned our stops meticulously, meeting every 10 miles for water, fuel, and essentials like sunscreen and ice. Each pit stop was to be a swift four minutes, just enough time to refuel without giving my muscles enough stationary time to have the chance to stiffen up. I had two different running vests, so when we met up, Dawn would help me swap out my vest for the new one that she'd fully stocked with ice water, electrolytes, and snacks.

My plan was to eat 200-300 calories per hour. This might sound like a lot, but the average runner burns between 60-100 calories per mile. Consuming all of the calories I was burning during a 50-mile race was going to be nearly impossible.

From miles 11-19, I was still feeling really good. This race was fun because there was something I had never seen before in a race. At that 20-mile mark, every runner had to get on a little boat in order to cross the intercoastal to a small island. Once there, we had to run a mile and a half around the exterior of the island, and then get back on the little boat in order to be transported back to the mainland. It was so different, so much fun, and definitely a highlight of the race for me.

The downside was that getting on the boat was tricky. It required jumping into calf-deep water before you could walk over to and climb into the waiting boat. Some people were stopping to take off their shoes, a lucky few had men on their crew who picked them up and

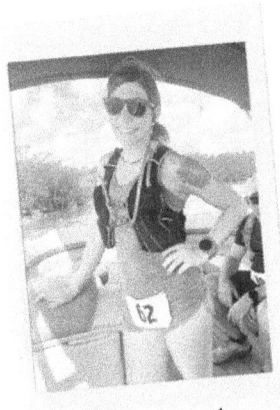

Mid-race boat ride

carried them to the boat so they wouldn't get their feet wet. At that moment I wished I'd thought ahead to have my husband there because I knew he would have gladly carried me, but he was at home with our son. I didn't want to waste the time taking off my shoes, so I chaotically jumped into the water even though I knew this meant that I'd have soaking wet socks and shoes for the mile and a half run around the island. While on my little boat ride, I was already texting Dawn to have a fresh pair of socks and shoes ready for me upon my return to the mainland. Luckily, I knew that I was well prepared, over prepared in fact, with 3 pairs of shoes and 5 pairs of socks just in case.

I was having so much fun and was feeling pretty good throughout the first half of the race. Once I reached about mile 25, that's when things started to heat up, *literally.* It was the hottest part of the day, and the sun was beating down with an unforgiving intensity. That great pace I'd been maintaining absolutely plummeted while the temperature soared into the mid-90s with barely a hint of shade. My mind started to spiral. How was I going to run in this harsh heat for another 25 miles? As much as I love the heat, (seriously, I'm a hot-weather runner, and dislike running in anything under 65°F) but the heat was seriously getting to me after hours and hours of running in it. I wasn't new to running in high temperatures, training in Miami often involved runs that left me drenched in sweat. I was well-prepared: drinking copious amounts of water, loading up on salt and electrolytes, and packing ice into my sports bra to keep cool. *I even paused to take a selfie and send it to my client, and now friend, Kelly, who had her own struggles with overheating during the Miami Marathon. I wanted her to know that she isn't the only runner that overheats and needs boob-ice.*

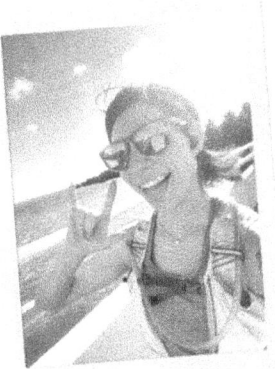

Boob-Ice for the win

Despite all my efforts, the heat wore me down and depleted my coolers of ice. Dawn even made an unplanned stop to purchase more! From miles 26 to 33, I walked more than I ran. The sun was beating down on me, and each step felt like it took all my strength. In desperation, I asked Dawn if she could run and pace me for the next few miles. Luckily, she had her running gear ready to go. I can't even begin to express how grateful I was that she was willing to be my crew AND pacer. Dawn's support was a lifeline. Having someone to share the journey with, to talk to, and to draw strength from, made all the difference in that miserable heat. She ended up accompanying me for 7 miles. While they

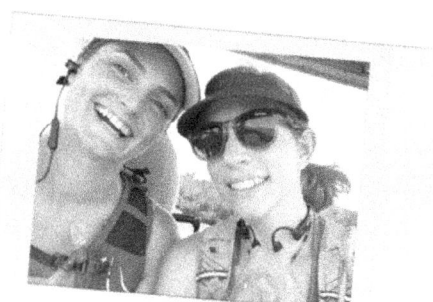

were the hottest, slowest, and most miserable, having her with me will forever be a core memory. We even stopped at a checkpoint for some cold watermelon that the race organizers provided us.

At the end of our 7 miles, she sprinted ahead to prepare my next hydration vest. When I caught up to her at our next meeting point, I was sure she was tired and exhausted herself. Rather than complain though, she rubbed petroleum jelly on my chafed skin, exchanged my hydration vest, and just held me when I needed a hug. In those moments, I realized how important it is to have a true support person throughout your race, not just someone who would refill supplies. She kept reminding me that I wasn't alone in this, that we were in it together.

Just like everything else in life, anything and everything is better when you have the right circle of people around you.

At mile 30, my body was starting to feel the fatigue from hours of insufficient calories. I was definitely not sticking to my 200-300 calorie per hour goal. Whether it was from the heat or just the excessive distance, my stomach was really upset, and the idea of eating anything at all was unappealing. This is a common issue amongst ultra runners because running such long distances diverts blood from the digestive tract to the working muscles, which can lead to having a messed-up tummy. With an amazing crew like Dawn, we anticipated this and planned ahead with a few ways to get me consuming more liquid calories. We had stashed some apple sauce and York peppermint patties in the cooler with ice. The cool applesauce felt good, and the ice was needed to keep the chocolate from melting in the heat. Peppermint patties not only soothed my stomach but also served as a symbolic treat, no longer provoking dark thoughts. They now represent my inner strength and how far I've come.

My feet and knees were also hurting quite a bit. After the boat ride and water crossing, I had switched into a pair of shoes that offered a lot of stability which I thought would be beneficial for the long distance. Unfortunately, they were also not as cushioned as some of my other shoes. The impact of pounding the ground for miles and miles with little to protect my joints was negatively impacting my body. We, again, went into problem solving mode. I was on this back road that wasn't easily accessible by car, and Dawn, too tired to run out and back to me, actually rode her bike to meet me at an unplanned mile marker so I could quickly change into a pair of shoes that was more cushioned and comfortable. *I guess I didn't over pack shoes after all.*

Around mile 35, a gift from the gods happened. A storm started to roll in, like a dark looming answer to my prayers. As soon as those black clouds appeared, the weather started to cool down, making the run considerably more manageable and enjoyable. Besides, I was riding that runner's high. This was the furthest I had ever run in a single go, and aside from being sore, I was feeling great again. I even found a few runners who were keeping the same pace I was comfortable with. Miles 35 to 42 were my fastest throughout the entire race in that overcast weather.

With the relief of the storm came the rain. I don't mind running in the rain. South Florida is known for its quick afternoon rain showers, and I'd enjoyed being caught running in more than a few. But then, lightning split the sky. I was still willing to brave the lightning. After all, I was riding my high and had less than 10 miles left of the race. But Dawn urged me to seek shelter in the car while the worst of the storm passed. I begged her to please let me keep going. We were running right along a main road at this point, so she drove a little way ahead of me in the car. As the next lightning bolt lit up the now darkened sky, Dawn counted, *"one-one-thousand, two-two thousand,"* BOOM thunder clapped. She insisted again, *"Please get in the car."* Very reluctantly, I agreed, even as my fortitude and drive screamed to keep going. When I first asked Dawn to be my crew, I promised that I would listen and follow her instructions regarding anything that had to do with my health and safety. And I knew that as an athlete and friend, I needed to follow through on my promises.

I sat in the car for what felt like eternity while the worst of the electrical storm raged outside. Those minutes in the car didn't feel like a welcome break, instead they were pure torture. All that energy and excitement for the race started to drain away as I stared out the window at the rain. I was wet and sitting in the car was making me cold. Dawn turned on the heat, but I could feel my muscles tightening up with every passing second.

I knew I had to get back out there, and when I stepped out of the car, I was sore, cold, and desperately hoping I would be able to find my groove again to push through the last few miles of the race. Even though the worst of the lightning had passed it was still pouring rain. Because I had known the day was going to be sweltering, I decided against packing a rain jacket. Sure, I knew there was a chance of rain, but I'd just thought that if it did rain, it would feel really good and cool me off. I was only partially correct: it did feel really good at first, and it did cool my core body temperature. The problem was that it had been so hot that my body had been working all day to cool itself down. Now with the rainstorm, my body was cooling down more than it needed to. During the final stages of the race, I had goosebumps and was shivering. My fingertips were going numb, and my body was actually in the beginning stages of hypothermia. *Hypothermia in July in South Florida, who would have thought of that?* Dawn. Dawn had thought of that, but I had laughed off her suggestion of packing a rescue blanket in the first aid kit. *Sorry Dawn.*

My mindset was tanking fast. Anyone who's run an Ultra Marathon will agree that success is about 40% skill, knowledge, and training, and 60% is mindset. Sitting in the car while the group I had been pacing with ran on and getting so cold took me out of the race, mentally. I was beyond relieved that I was almost done, and before I knew it, I'd crossed the finish line. It was anti-climactic though, and honestly, I was just thankful to be able to have a towel around me and to sit down. Every marathon I'd participated in before had ended with celebration, excitement, my arms flung out and flying across the finish line. But this race, when it ended, it was just over. I didn't necessarily feel any huge sense of pride that I had just run a whole 50 miles in one go.

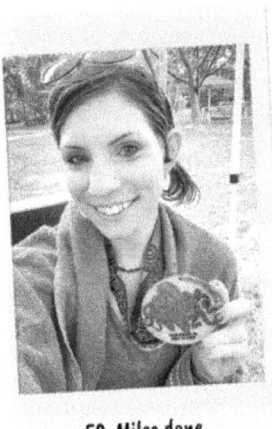

50-Miles done

Looking back now, I understand why this race felt different. I had lost that connection, that momentum, and because I was so close to the end when the storm hit, I didn't have a chance to regain that excitement before crossing the finish line. I was so upset and frustrated because before the rain, and that terrible time spent sitting in the car, my body had felt so good! I was proud of my body for carrying me so far, I could have finished stronger, and maybe I could have even run further if not for the lightning, the time in the car, and the rain cooling me off too much. Maybe if I only had to endure one of the three, I still could have. All those things together created the perfect storm to take my mind out of the race and caused my body to give in before the finish line.

Rather than risk either of us being uncomfortable with her crewing me again, Dawn and I came to an agreement for any future races she crews me for: She'll cheer me on and keep me as hydrated and fed as she can. She'll keep me as safe as she can when it comes to everything but lightning. I'm responsible for making my own call when it comes to lighting . . . and I will listen to her the first time she tells me to do something during a race, even if I don't want to. That includes packing a rain jacket and rescue blanket.

Regardless of the weather and that struggle at the end, the 50-mile race was an amazing experience. It made me feel much better about the Spartan Ultra Championships that were coming up. I felt like I was ready for the 24-hour obstacle race, I was mentally and physically prepared for almost anything.

The countdown was on. The Spartan Ultra World Championships were now just weeks away, and once I was warmed up and dry, I was the strongest I had ever been.

But then, something no one could have predicted changed everything.

The fires that had been burning in California started getting out of control. Rumors started to circulate that they were bad enough that it might actually affect the race that was scheduled in Lake Tahoe. That entire week was rough. I literally had the local California news streaming on my computer 24/7, checking for updates every few minutes, hoping for a miracle.

The fires kept spreading, and even though they were still miles away from the actual location of the race, thick smoke filled the sky, causing the air quality to plummet. The toxic, dangerous air conditions continued to get worse throughout the week, and just two days before my husband and I were set to board our flight, the Spartan race directors officially decided to call off the World Championships.

Ally Robinson

Oh BABY

Getting the news that the Spartan Ultra World Championships were canceled was like a punch to the gut, a cruel twist of fate that left me reeling. All those hours, the endless miles, the sweat, and the sacrifice—it felt like it was all for nothing. I had poured my heart and soul into training for this race. While the fires burned, I held on to so much hope that the fires would be contained that when the call was finally made to cancel the race, I literally cried. The grief was overwhelming, like mourning the death of a dream. It felt like a piece of me had been ripped away.

In the days that followed, I was a mess. I stopped training, something I had never imagined doing. I slept in, skipping my usual morning runs. The structure and discipline that had defined my days fell apart. My motivation was shattered, and I felt lost without the goal that had been driving me forward the last couple of months.

For my own mental health, I needed to step back, to give myself permission to grieve the loss of this dream. My body, weary from relentless training, welcomed the rest. I allowed myself to slow down.

When I was finally ready to resume running. I did so for my soul. No training plan, not to chase a goal but to soothe my spirit. These runs were different. They weren't about speed or endurance; they were about finding peace.

I could feel that familiar darkness starting to creep back into my life. But this time, I had the tools I needed to find peace. Running had become not only a hobby and my career but also a coping mechanism, one of the most important tools in my kit to keep me from going back to those dark places. The slower pace allowed me to reflect and to reconnect with my love for running.

It was nice to slow down. I had been training so hard for so long that I had forgotten what it was like to just enjoy regular life. There was a life outside of the gym, long runs, and the treadmill. I spent more time with my son and husband, reconnecting in ways I hadn't realized I had been missing. It was a gift to reconnect with the ordinary joys of life and to remember that there was a world beyond the gym.

I began to appreciate the small things again——morning coffee with my husband instead of waking up before the sun for long workouts. I took my son to the park and spent more time running around with him instead of being so sore I could hardly move. This time away from rigorous training was a reminder that balance is essential.

At the end of October, me and my little brother, Logan who is now 16 and towers over me in height, were preparing for our annual half marathon. A tradition that we've been doing for the last couple of years. He ran track at his high school, so it was a great way for us to bond over running and training sessions and share the excitement of race day.

The night before the race, I tried to go to bed early, but my mind was restless, swirling with thoughts. Since my days of terrible nightmares, I haven't been much of a dreamer. But on the rare occasion that I do have dreams, they can be wild and vivid. On this night in particular, I dreamed that I took a pregnancy test… and it was… positive.

When my alarm went off at 4 a.m., I kept thinking about the dream. Could it be true? I rummaged through my bathroom cabinet and found an old pregnancy test that I had tucked away. With trembling hands, I took the test, watching breathlessly as the faintest pink line appeared. My heart raced. Was it real? Was this just a trick of my tired, wishful eyes?

I continued getting ready for the race, but my mind was a spinning whirlwind of emotions. *Could I really be pregnant?* My husband and I had always dreamed of expanding our family. I mean, we were content with our little family of three, but there was always something in the back of both of our minds saying that we weren't yet a complete family unit. But, having a baby is a big deal, a huge commitment, and it never seemed like a good time, especially when I was so invested in growing both as an athlete and an online business owner.

Yet, once again, I learned that life has a way of unfolding in mysterious and beautiful ways. Despite the lingering heartache I felt from missing out on experiencing the Spartan World Championships, those two little faint pink lines brought a light to my life, a sense of promise that filled my heart with joy.

On the drive to the race, I turned to my little brother, showing him the test that I'd stuffed into my pocket. *"You see two pink lines, right?"* He confirmed my suspicions. I was indeed pregnant, and not just seeing things. Of course, as a running coach, I *would* find out that I was pregnant the morning before running a half marathon, in a gingerbread man costume, no less. *(Hey, it was a Halloween-themed race, and if you don't think it's hilarious for a running coach to be dressed like a childhood storybook character whose claim to fame is shouting, "Run run as fast as you can, you can't catch me," then you're crazy.)* I was on cloud nine! It was as if the universe had given me a runner's high before the race began. I couldn't wait to go home and tell my husband. *(Yes, you read that right. My little brother knew I was expecting before my husband did. What can I say? Race days can be chaotic.)*

We knew that out of all the half-marathons Logan, and I ran together, this would probably be the slowest. He was nursing a sore knee, and now all throughout the race, my thoughts kept drifting back to those two little pink lines and the tiny life growing inside me. I whispered to my unborn baby, *"This is our first of many adventures together."* My brother and I took the race slow and enjoyed running along the boardwalk of Miami Beach. As we approached the final stretch of the race, in tradition, we clasped hands and crossed the finish line victoriously together.

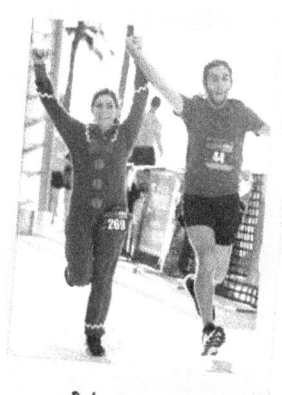

Baby On Board

Back home, I could hardly contain my excitement as I shared the news with my husband. The look of pure joy on his face was priceless. We spent the rest of the afternoon talking about our growing family, imagining the exciting life changes that were about to start happening.

Later in the evening, we had another reason to celebrate: the grand opening party of Donny's motorcycle shop. On the way to the shop to set up for the party, he stopped at the liquor store to purchase an expensive bottle of whiskey. As the event began, the showroom looked amazing, the bikes Donny customized with performance enhanced engines sat on display. As the night progressed, the shop filled with music, friends, and fellow motorcycle enthusiasts, all there to support Donny in his new venture.

At the end of the night, as the party wound down, Donny gathered everyone around for one final toast with the whiskey he'd purchased. With his closest buddies and supporters by his side, he raised his glass for one last celebratory shot, as he proudly announced that he was going to be a dad, *again.* Although there may be unspoken rules about when to announce a pregnancy, it felt special to share such exciting news at such an exciting time.

I knew deep in my soul that our baby would be a little girl. My husband and I calculated the estimated due date, sometime around the end of June or early July, and we knew right away that her name was Summer. The name seemed to encapsulate all the warmth and fun that this new chapter in our lives held.

This metaphorical roller coaster ride reminded me that even in the darkest moments of life, when it feels like everything you've worked for is being taken away, life has a way of surprising us, offering new beginnings and unexpected glimmers of joy. Sure, my plans took a wild turn. Hell, I was supposed to be running an Ultra World Championship in Tahoe, not sitting back in Miami talking with my husband about how we were going to rearrange the house to make room for a new baby. This was a 9-month plus long ultra that I had definitely not trained for, but I was ready for it.

Running while pregnant is a wild ride. The first 12 weeks felt like I was carrying the weight of the world, even before my baby bump started to show. I was tired all the time. Just putting on my running clothes to head out for a run was exhausting. Every morning, I battled fatigue that seemed to seep into my bones. But I kept pushing through because, as a running coach, I felt like I needed to keep striving to be that inspirational pregnant running momma, continuing to expand on the narrative that pregnancy is not a disability, and you can keep running and crossing finish lines even with a bun in the oven.

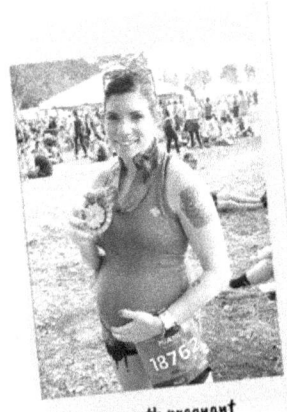

6-month pregnant
half-marathon

Originally, I had my heart set on running the Miami Marathon again that January. I would only be about 6 months pregnant so that seemed doable. But with the relentless exhaustion weighing me down, I knew my body was sending me a clear message: *slow down.* Listening to that inner voice was tough, but necessary. In the best interest of my growing, tired body I made the call to drop down to the half marathon. And, at the halfway point, as the full marathoners veered off to tackle the grueling second half, we (my baby bump and I) confidently split off. It was the first time I embraced the shorter half distance not as a failure but as a smart calculated decision.

Throughout my pregnancy, I ran multiple half marathons and even a Spartan Beast (granted, it was the non-competitive wave, and I had to skip a few obstacles, but it was a victory in itself). These races weren't about setting personal records or pushing my limits. *I actually had to stop a few times throughout these races to pee because my plus one was sitting on my bladder.* These races were about proving to myself that I could adapt and still find joy in the sport I loved. I remember the first time I felt her kick while I was preparing for a run. It was like she was cheering me on, reminding me that we were in this together.

At around 25 weeks into my pregnancy, I failed my glucose test and ended up needing to make some drastic changes to my diet, to manage my blood sugars for the rest of my pregnancy. Around 30 weeks my blood pressure started to rise, and I was getting migraine headaches daily, I felt terrible. My OB made the call that I should stop running for the rest of my pregnancy. Just as I had promised Dawn that I'd listen to her regarding my health, I had to give my doctor the same respect. As much as I didn't want it to, the active, race-filled pregnancy I had envisioned for myself was quickly slipping away.

I gradually realized how much I used running as a band-aid for my mental and emotional health. Running became my escape, my therapy, and my way of coping with life's challenges. When my doctor told me to stop running during my pregnancy due to health concerns, it felt like my entire identity was stripped away. Sure, I was still allowed to do prenatal yoga and daily walks, but IT'S NOT THE SAME! I was lost without my routine runs, the one thing that kept me grounded and sane. The absence of running forced me to confront my emotions and mental health head-on. It was a difficult and painful realization that maybe I wasn't as recovered and stable as I thought. Ultimately, while running is still an amazing tool, it taught me the importance of addressing the underlying issues rather than just masking them with miles.

6 weeks later, my doctor made the call that it was in the best interest of me and the baby to deliver as soon as possible. We ended up scheduling a cesarean a full month earlier than planned. I had a c-section with my son previously, so I knew what to expect. But it's scary going into any operation room, plus the added fears around having a baby early. When I heard my daughter's first cry, all the fear and doubt melted away. She was here, and she was perfect. Our little Summer baby just so happened to be born on a rainy Spring day.

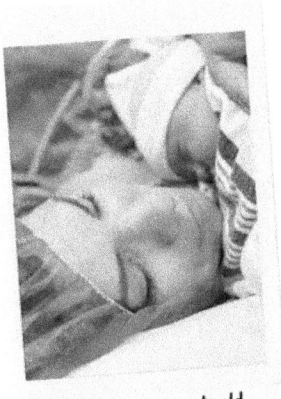

Only a few moments old

After delivering Summer, the journey back to running was a slow one. The recovery from this c-section took much longer than the first. I tried to rest as much as possible, but my legs were itching to get moving. One of the big purchases I made while I was pregnant was a heavy duty all terrain jogging stroller. A couple of weeks postpartum, I took the new stroller for a test run, well, walk. It was slow, but I felt so much gratitude to be able to move freely with minimal pain.

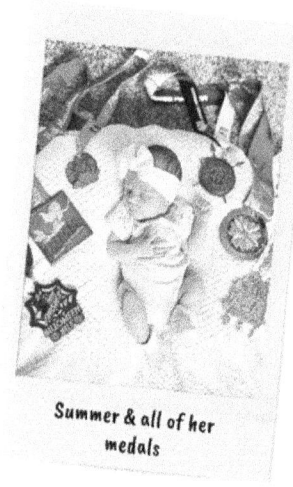

Summer & all of her
medals

I probably could have started running sooner, but I knew the importance of letting my body fully heal before jumping back into intense exercise. So, I focused on what I could do. After having my daughter, I experienced a separation between my abdominal muscles, *diastasis recti*, which is common in pregnancy and postpartum, but can make engaging your core difficult and even cause urinary incontinence. So, once I was given approval by my doctor I started working on diaphragmatic breathing exercises. I also started working on my pelvic floor muscles, basically doing Kegels. I laughed and told my physical therapist that because both of my babies had been delivered via c-section, with neither of them coming out my who-ha, my vaginal muscles were just fine. *This was one of those times when I needed to realize I didn't know everything.* They explained that it's all connected down there the pelvic floor and deep core. And yes, I did, in fact, still need to work on those strengthening those Kegel muscles.

Eventually, I could start including more core exercises like dead bugs, glute bridges, and side planks. It might not be super cool or glamorous, but this is what I focused on for the first few months of Summer's life. I'd set her on the floor for tummy time, and she would watch me do my breathing and pelvic exercises. I did not rush the process; I just focused on building a strong foundation (and core) so that I would be in the best possible position when I started running again.

At 12 weeks postpartum, I laced up my shoes and went for my first run, feeling a mixture of excitement and trepidation. My body felt different than it had before, more feeble and less agile than I remembered. The first few minutes were tough, my muscles protesting the sudden activity after months of a different kind of exertion. It wasn't much better than my very first run ever—awkward, slow, and I was out of breath within just a few minutes.

I started with super-short interval runs and gradually extended the length of those runs and intervals. I couldn't worry about my speed, instead I was focused on my heartrate, breathing, and running form, as well as building back up my endurance. I was running the same trail along the beach that I had when I was training at the peak of my running career. It was a trying experience to cross paths with people I used to run with before, to see them going so much faster than I was, running races that I wasn't. I had to check my ego at the door and get comfortable with the fact that once again, this was my race, at my pace, and now, I was doing it with a jogging stroller. It's one thing to coach about getting into running, building endurance, and getting faster, it's another thing to actually demonstrate those skills, modeling for my clients exactly how it's done.

Despite all the experience and coaching under my belt, starting over wasn't easy. I had to let go of the expectations I once had for myself, the speed and endurance that used to come effortlessly. Instead, I embraced where I was now, celebrating every mile, every small victory. My first continuous postpartum 5k? I shouted *"YES!"* with a sense of triumph. My first 10k? I cheered *"YAY!"* And when I finally ran my first sub-30 minute 3 miles after giving birth, I pumped my fists in the air, and celebrated as if I just set a new PR or qualified for the Olympic trials.

As I tell my clients all the time, you aren't starting over from the beginning; you are starting over with experience. You're starting over, armed with all of the lessons and resilience you've built along the way. It's about using your knowledge and experience as a foundation to build something even stronger.

One of the hardest parts about getting back into running was finding the time to do it. Not only did I have my son, who's active and loves being the center of my world, and my audacious self-decided I didn't need a maternity leave from my business, so I still had client calls and training plans to write, but now I had a baby girl as well, who needed naps, and feedings, and snuggles. Finding the motivation to keep going was tough. I remember mornings when the last thing I wanted to do was lace up my shoes and go for a run. The weight of sleepless nights, the constant demands of motherhood, and the pressure of keeping my business afloat felt like too much. But every time I pushed through, I felt a little stronger, a little more like myself.

Gradually, I rebuilt my strength. And got back to my normally scheduled running. Only this time I was pushing a stroller for most of my miles. Running with Summer became our special time together. Her laughter and curious eyes as we explored new trails brought a new kind of joy to my runs. She was my little cheerleader, and with every giggle and smile, I felt more motivated to keep going.

Ally Robinson

Strong is the New Skinny

After my hard pregnancy I felt like my body had betrayed me. Here I was, a young, healthy athlete, and yet my body hadn't been able to handle something as natural as having a baby, without complications. There were days when I would look in the mirror and barely recognize the person staring back at me. The physical changes from pregnancy, the scars from surgery, the exhaustion etched into my face. But then I realized how much my body had actually handled. I'd grown two humans, I'd run marathons, jumped over 8-foot walls, climbed ropes, run 50-mile races, earned more medals than I can count, and survived my own attempt to take my life. It was hard not to appreciate my body when I started making that list. I was so thankful to be in that mindset now, but it wasn't always like that.

As a child, teenager, and young adult, I struggled with my body image. Skinny was never skinny enough. Even as a 95-pound ballerina, I believed I'd be more talented, more likable, and prettier if I could just shed a few more pounds. Despite being objectively thin, I fixated on that tiny bit of fat spilling over my bathing suit or the skin I could pinch when I sat down. So many times, as a young girl, I held scissors to my stomach, wishing I could just cut it off. I thought that if I was just thinner, I would be more successful. I felt like I wasn't good enough and that I would have to change who I was in order to be accepted. I was constantly comparing myself to others and I was feeling horribly inadequate.

In middle school it was brought to light that I was skipping lunch. They even made me talk to the school counselor. My mom saw me eat dinner every night. She saw me eat and indulge in sweets in the evening. But in my mind, I was allowed to eat those foods because I had starved myself throughout the day, skipping breakfast and lunch.

They all thought it was a plea for attention, and I was okay with that assumption. It kept them from suspecting the deeper issues at play. To throw them off further, I exaggerated my fear of vomiting, making it seem impossible that I could ever force myself to throw up. It was during summer break when I made myself purge my food for the first time.

Being home with my mom all day I couldn't just not eat. So, I would eat as normal and as soon as she left the house to get groceries or run errands I would run upstairs to the bathroom. I'd turn the sink or shower on high to muffle the sound and use my toothbrush to make myself sick.

It felt like I had discovered a life hack: I could eat whatever I wanted and then just purge it. When I nearly got caught, I pretended to be sick, and no one questioned it. This pattern continued throughout my teenage years, especially during times when I felt particularly inadequate or self-conscious. Choosing hobbies like ballet and then getting into modeling didn't help my desire to be thin or improve my body image.

It wasn't until I was pregnant with my son that my disordered eating habits started to change. Throwing up by choice was one thing. Throwing up from severe morning sickness was another. For the first time, I couldn't control the nausea and vomiting. I remember lying in bed crying because I was so hungry, but I could barely hold down water and saltine crackers. The first trimester was brutal, but when the morning sickness finally subsided, I could eat normally again. Actually, I could gorge myself without fear. With a baby growing inside of me, I wasn't worried about gaining weight. In fact, I loved watching my body change and my belly grow. Donny was amazed when I could suddenly devour half a pizza, whereas previously, I would only nibble a couple of bites and claim to be full.

During my pregnancy with Kylo, I gained 55 pounds. That's right, I gained over half my original body weight! At just 5 feet tall, I was all belly, and my petite frame bore the weight of my growing baby with a kind of confidence that I had never felt before.

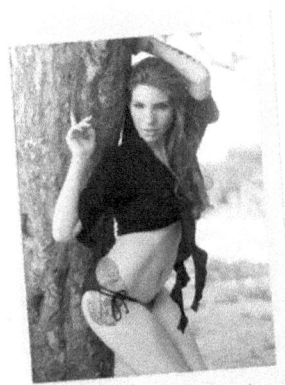

Modeling photo 2.5 months after my first baby

Once my son was born though, my postpartum body mortified me. I immediately wanted to revert back to my old ways. But I couldn't. Because now I *actually* had this new aversion for throwing up, I decided to severely cut back on calories. Maybe it was my young age combined with my extremely low-calorie diet, allowing me to "bounce back" to my pre-motherhood body fairly quickly. I scheduled a photoshoot only 10 weeks after giving birth as motivation to lose the baby weight as quickly as possible. Two and a half months after giving birth, I was on the beach in a skimpy outfit, looking as though I had never been pregnant, outside of my now weirdly misshapen belly button.

This rapid weight loss that photographers applauded me for came at a cost. I struggled to produce breast milk. I desperately wanted to nourish my son naturally, but my body couldn't keep up with his nutritional needs while I wasn't allowing myself to receive proper nutrition. This failure to successfully breastfeed only deepened my feelings of inadequacy, as a mother. *How could I be a good mom to Kylo if I couldn't even feed him?*

When I started running, I had no concept of what *good nutrition* was. I had no idea how to actually nourish my body, which probably added to the struggle of those early days. Malnutrition certainly did not help with injury prevention. I thought that eating less was the key to being thin and healthy, but I quickly learned that it was quite the opposite. My diet lacked balance, and my body was constantly deprived of the nutrients it needed to perform and recover.

After my first marathon, when I was determined to become healthier and fitter, I had to learn about macros, calories, and the quality of the food I was eating. I started educating myself, reading books, consulting with nutritionists, and experimenting with different foods. I actually ended up gaining a few pounds, but man, did I feel so much better! I mean, I could actually carry groceries up to our second-story apartment without being winded. My energy levels soared, and my overall well-being improved dramatically.

Learning to cook *healthy* meals that tasted good was a game-changer. I discovered that fueling my body didn't mean sacrificing flavor or enjoyment. I began experimenting with recipes, using fresh, whole ingredients, and finding creative ways to make nutritious meals delicious.

As I became stronger and faster, I started to see my body in a new light. I began to appreciate my body for what it could do rather than how small it could be. This shift in perspective was liberating. I realized that confidence comes from valuing our body's capabilities, not just its appearance. Because the truth is, no matter how skinny I became, it was never skinny enough. There was always a new standard to chase, a new flaw to fixate on.

Embracing this new mindset wasn't easy and didn't happen overnight. I had to unlearn years of ingrained behaviors and beliefs about my body. There were days when I would catch myself slipping back into old habits, scrutinizing my reflection with a critical eye. But each time, I reminded myself of the incredible things my body had done and continued to do. I reminded myself that my worth wasn't tied to a number on the scale or the size of my clothes.

When I started coaching women to reach their running goals, I was astounded by how many of them started running later in life as a way to lose weight and get healthier. Many were following restrictive diets, completely removing vital food groups, or severely cutting calories. I saw so much of my younger self in them, and I knew I had to help them make a change. I pledged to educate these women on how to fuel their bodies properly and to emphasize the importance of proper nutrition and self-care. How to have a better relationship with food and fitness. I wanted to show them how to lose weight in a sustainable way that would allow them to have the energy to crush their health and fitness goals both now and in the long-term.

I challenged my clients to shift their focus away from the number they saw on their scale and concentrate on consuming more of the good foods and moving their bodies more by doing activities they enjoyed. By doing that, my clients wound up feeling better about themselves, their bodies, and what their bodies could do. The most amazing thing was that these women still wound up losing weight, and it was happening easier and faster than they'd expected. Once I realized that what I was offering was working for other women, I decided to take my newfound message and passion to my Facebook group. My goal was, and still is, to start a worldwide movement encouraging more and more women around the world to fall in love with their bodies, feel great, and achieve their running goals.

Seven years later, when I got pregnant with my daughter, I was determined to approach things differently than I had during and after my first pregnancy. This time, I wanted to live and demonstrate my teachings to my clients. I committed to eating a balanced diet throughout my pregnancy and focused on nourishing foods that would benefit both me and my growing baby.

After Summer was born, I took a gradual approach to losing the excess weight, inviting my clients to join me on this journey. I shared my experiences, struggles, and victories with them, focusing on the importance of nourishing our bodies rather than chasing rapid weight loss. It wasn't about quick fixes; it was about long-term health and sustainability.

I filled my plate with fruits, veggies, and complex carbs. I also made sure to drink plenty of water to support breastfeeding. And it worked. I was able to breastfeed my daughter for much longer than I had my son, and that little accomplishment made me incredibly proud. My healthy eating habits weren't just nourishing me; they were sustaining her too.

One Bad Mother Runner

When Kylo was 3 years old he looked at me with those big, excited eyes and said, *"Mommy, I want a medal. I want to win a race like you."* His words made me pause. Could he really be ready for a race?

After much thought and consideration, my husband and I decided there was no harm in letting him participate in a 5k. We even brought the stroller, but my son insisted, full of confidence, that he wanted to run. I was worried for so many reasons. My son has my competitiveness. He could feel defeated when others passed us by. He might be heartbroken when we did not ACTUALLY win the race.

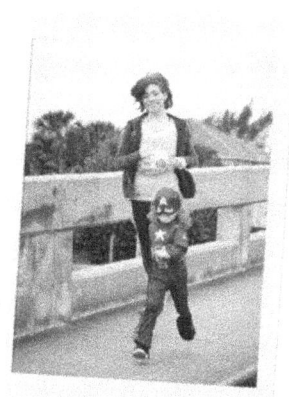

When we lined up at the start of the race, my son eagerly made friends with all the adults around him. It was October, nearing Halloween and he opted to wear his Captain America costume. *He swore that it would make him run faster.*

Kylo 'winning' the race

"I'm gonna win." "I'm gonna run really fast like mommy." "I'm gonna get a medal." He declared proudly to everyone around us.

When the race started, my son ran forward, full steam ahead! Obviously, his energy and speed quickly burned out. He said, *"Mommy, I'm gonna walk until my legs refuel."* Then, two minutes later, he was off on a sprint again. Around the 2-mile mark, he finally accepted a piggyback ride from me, but only so his legs could *refuel faster.* Before I knew it, he was off on another sprint.

As we went on, we fell further behind the other runners. My worries came rushing back. *What if the finish line was gone by the time we got there? What if there was no one cheering? What if there were no more medals?* But as we neared the end, I saw the finish line still standing, with two volunteers holding medals.

As we approached, the volunteers erupted in cheers. They hooped and hollered with all the enthusiasm they could muster as my little toddler went full speed toward the finish line.

When the volunteers handed him his medal, I held my breath, bracing for his reaction.

And right on cue, my son started to jump, shout, and cheer!

"I won!" "I won the race!" "I'm the fastest ever!"

It was a moment of pure joy. My 3-year-old had just run three miles and finished with the biggest smile, not caring one bit about not being the first to cross the finish line.

In that proud mom moment, he reminded me of a valuable lesson: it's not always about coming in first. It's about running your race, in your way, and finding joy in every step of the journey, that's the true win!

Over the years, my son has only run a handful of races with me. I treasure those memories. I love that he wants to run with me sometimes, but I also respect that running isn't necessarily his hobby or interest. Kylo has his own unique passions and talents, and I celebrate those just as enthusiastically as I focus on my own. Kylo has always been extremely artistic and would, most of the time, rather be inside drawing, painting, or writing stories. I marvel at his creativity and encourage him every chance I get, even enrolling him in an art club at his school and additional art classes over the summer break. I can already picture a future where I'm walking through galleries filled with his artwork or reading his published books.

As for Summer, I am excited to see what passions and dreams she will develop as she grows older. Whether she wants to run, paint, dance, or explore something entirely different, I am committed to supporting her every step of the way. As her mother, I want to be her biggest cheerleader, just as I am for Kylo.

I used to worry about how my running might be taking time away from my family and my responsibilities as a mom. There were times I felt guilty, wondering if I was being selfish by dedicating so many hours to training and races. But then Kylo started to show genuine excitement about my achievements. He even brags to his friends at school about the medals hanging on my wall. It's in those moments that I realize that I am not just running for myself—I am running for my children, too.

By pursuing my passion for running, I've been able to model for Kylo and Summer that it's okay to have interests outside of being a mom. I'm proud to have shown them both that it's possible to be a loving and involved mother and still pursue my own dreams outside of raising a family. While I hope Kylo remembers this as he grows older and maybe starts a family of his own, it's particularly important to me that Summer carries this message with her into adulthood.

I don't want my daughter to grow up feeling like if she one day has children that her dreams and goals have to take a backseat. When our daughters see us chasing our dreams—whether it's running a marathon, building a career, or simply taking time to enjoy a hobby—they learn that it's okay to have ambitions. They see that it's possible to be an amazing mom AND still pursue personal goals. This will empower them to dream big and go after what they want in life.

There's something incredibly powerful about setting and achieving goals. Crossing the finish line of a race, landing a new job, or mastering a new skill shows our kids what's possible when we believe in ourselves. They need to know they can do the same. By sharing our successes and even our failures, we teach them that it's okay to take risks and that every step, even the occasional misstep, is part of the journey.

Growing up, I watched my mom dedicate every ounce of her being to raising us. She put her dreams, desires, and ambitions on hold, focusing solely on our needs and ensuring that her kids had the best possible upbringing. Her days were filled with our activities, our lives, leaving little room for her own. She was always there for us—at every school event, every doctor appointment, every dance recital. But in doing so, she quietly set aside her own passions and aspirations. I am incredibly grateful to have had such a loving mother while I was growing up. Her sacrifices shaped my childhood. The choices she made allowed me and my siblings to have so many amazing memories. We went on family vacations, had grand birthday parties, and experienced extravagant Christmas mornings, all because she made it possible. I always saw my mom working tirelessly to keep up with the house, raise us kids, and take care of my sick sister. She even acted as both mom and dad while he was gone at work or preoccupied with other things. She did all of this when I knew that what she really wanted was to get her own photography business off the ground and maybe not rely so much on my dad for financial support.

Now, years later, my mom is in her 50s and transitioning into having an empty nest as Logan heads off to college. I see her working hard to rediscover herself and who she is. It's as though she's peeling back layers of herself that had been hidden for years, unearthing dreams that were long buried. I see her growing as a woman, standing up for herself, especially after separating from my father.

I can't help but wish that she had been able to model that strength and self-fulfillment for my siblings and me as we were growing up. I would have benefited from seeing her as a strong female role model.

Watching my mom bravely step into this new chapter of her life has shown me that reinvention is possible at any age. It's never too late to become the person you were always meant to be.

As a young adult struggling to find myself, I didn't have the role models I desperately needed. I had no idea what a strong woman who stood up for herself looked like. I had never had an example of a healthy relationship. I had to expand my circle of women. I had to seek out women in healthy marriages. I had to find women who were building businesses and changing the world. I joined groups, attended workshops, and surrounded myself with women who embodied the things I wanted to see in myself.

Ultimately, I had to become the role model that I needed as a child.

I am by no means a perfect mom, and I do not have everything figured out. What I do know is that our kids are always watching and listening. Kylo used to ask me every day if I'd had my coffee yet. My response was always the same, *"yes, Kylo, I've had my coffee."* Finally, after more than a few days of this back and forth, I asked him why he was so concerned about my coffee consumption. *"Because mom, without your coffee, you'll die."* I realized that I must have made some offhand remark while Kylo was within listening range about how *I NEEDED coffee, or I'd die*. Kylo took this quite literally and was very concerned for my life.

It's not just what we say. As a runner and a mom, I've also found that the way we live our lives can have a huge impact on our children. They're always watching, absorbing, and learning from us, whether we realize it or not. I remember one time my son said, *"When I am an adult, I am going to eat orange potatoes."* I know he means sweet potatoes. *"Oh yeah? Why is that?"* *"Because you eat orange potatoes, and you run really fast. When I'm a grown-up, I want to run fast too."* It makes me laugh thinking about it. I don't recall ever saying anything about eating sweet potatoes, or that they're helping me to run fast. He made that connection completely by himself. It's amazing what kids observe and pick up on. When we choose healthy foods, we're not just taking care of ourselves; we're setting a positive example for our children. They may not choose to participate in the sweet potato eating now, but they're more likely to do so when they get older.

Our kids notice our habits and behaviors, even when we're not consciously teaching them. Sometimes especially when we're not trying to teach them! When we choose healthy foods and live active lives, we're setting a positive example for our children. *With that in mind, what are we doing to be role models for our kids?* I often find myself thinking about the lessons my children are teaching me in return.

One afternoon, when my daughter was 8 months old, I placed her in front of the mirror. Summer was completely fascinated by her own reflection. Her eyes were wide with excitement and love, free from any judgment. Watching my daughter gaze at herself with pure wonder made me think. *Kids don't see flaws or imperfections.* So, when did we, as women, start being so hard on ourselves? When did we begin picking apart our reflections?

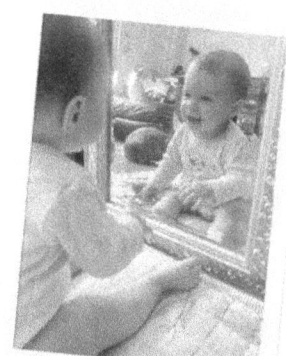

Summer, falling in love with what she saw in the mirror

Babies and young kids are unapologetically themselves. They express their emotions freely, without a second thought about what others might think. If they're happy, they laugh with abandon. If they're sad, they cry without shame. They don't hide their feelings or pretend to be something they're not. This kind of authenticity is something we tend to lose as we grow up. I'm not suggesting we should revert to throwing tantrums or acting out our frustrations like toddlers, but perhaps we could learn to be a bit more open and genuine in expressing our emotions and needs. I know I still struggle with opening up about how I am feeling. I bottle things up until I can't contain it anymore, and it explodes in a blaze of anger or into a week-long depressive episode. Maybe that's why I love those long grueling races. I can't mask my emotions when I'm hours into a race.

I laugh, remembering when my son was about three years old. He got so attached to his Halloween costume that he wouldn't take it off long after October was over. He wore it to his first 5k race, to the park, and even to the grocery store. People would give him funny looks or make comments, but he didn't care. He was just so happy and proud of his costume. It reminds me to be more of my authentic self, maybe that's why I dye my hair a bright magenta color or why pink is such a big part of my brand. It reminds me of the days of pink sequined skirts, back when I was my true self, before I was worried about the opinions of others.

Children also possess an incredible sense of wonder. They find joy in discovering new things, whether it's the texture of a leaf, the sound of a bird, or the taste of a new food. This curiosity drives their learning and growth. As adults, we often lose this sense of wonder, getting stuck in our routines and daily grind. Rediscovering our curiosity can bring back some of that excitement for life. I remember the first time I took my son to Disney World, and I saw the magic of Disney once again through the eyes of a child. I want to see life like that all the time, not just in anticipation of a race or a glorious vacation, but to see the beauty of the day-to-day and the bits of magic it holds.

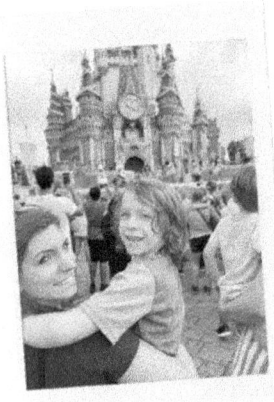

The magic of Disney

Every child is unique and progresses at their own pace. Kylo, for instance, was a remarkably fast learner, even as a baby. He quickly picked up his first words, gestures, and common commands well before the suggested milestone windows. His rapid development continued with physical milestones; he was crawling and walking ahead of schedule, taking his first steps before 11 months. Toddling around, Kylo was determined to explore the world on his own terms.

When Summer was born, I expected a similar pattern. I diligently checked all the milestone charts, anticipating that same swift progression. But her pace of growth was different, it took her longer to hit the same milestones Kylo had easily surpassed. From sitting to cruising to walking, she did it all in her own time. Yet, I was full of so much anxiety and worry that my baby wasn't excelling. There was nothing wrong with her; she simply had her own pace. The experience brought to mind the same lesson I had to learn. Stay in my own lane.

If I hadn't had Kylo to compare with, I might not have noticed that Summer was slower to pick up certain skills. But that comparison was unnecessary and unfair to her. It's okay if the journey takes longer; it doesn't mean there is anything wrong with the progress being made. And there definitely doesn't need to be any comparison to others along the way.

Speaking of little ones walking, watching a toddler take their first steps is absolutely fascinating. They embody fearlessness and tenacity, taking these qualities to a whole new level. They don't worry about failing; they embrace the process of learning with pure determination. Watching Summer learn to walk is a perfect example. She stumbles, falls, and gets back up. What a great metaphor and lesson for the grandness of this thing called life.

Gosh, it's just fascinating how many life lessons happen in the mundane of life. One of my many goals in life is to never stop learning, exploring, and absorbing these tidbits of knowledge that happen in this never-ending race.

Dear Ally

I wish I could travel back in time and visit my younger self. I would show her the woman she would one day grow up to be. Or at least write her a letter and tell her all the wonderful things that will one day be her new normal. It would go something like this.

Dear 15-year-old Ally,

I know right now things feel pretty rough, I know that heartache you feel. I am so proud of you for waking up this morning. I know it took every ounce of strength you have, but guess what? You did it! It's hard to see it now, but there's a really good reason you're still here, and it's worth sticking around to find out what it is.

I know you're feeling pretty broken right now and maybe even a bit unlovable. But hold on—things are about to change in the best way. There is a time in the not too distant future when you'll be in a safe space. You will heal and rebuild yourself, much like the Japanese art of Kintsugi, where broken pottery is fixed with gold, making it even more beautiful than before.

Your broken pieces will be held together with the lessons and love that you've accumulated on your journey.

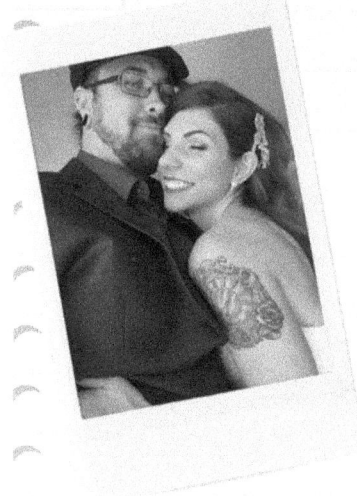

One day, you're going to wake up next to your absolute favorite person. Yes, Ally, your adoring husband, your life partner! This person will see you, not just look at the surface level, he'll truly see you—flaws, quirks, and all—and think you're amazing. Some people wait a lifetime to meet their soulmate, but you only have a few more years to go. And when you do, you'll understand why you had to endure so much heartbreak. While I wouldn't normally advise anyone to marry the person they meet at 19 years old, I can confidently tell you that a decade later, your marriage will still be strong and thriving, a testament to the love and partnership you've built together.

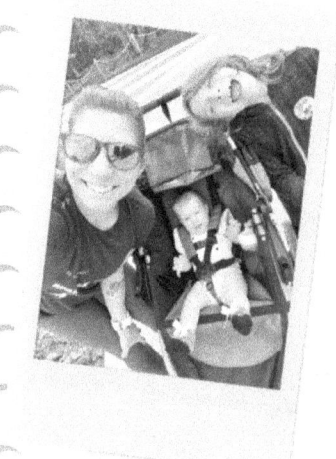

Your beautiful daughter, a tiny bundle of sass and sweetness, will be sleeping peacefully in her crib next to your bed. And then, there's your son. Your rambunctious 8-year-old boy, who will come bounding into your room, full of life and energy, seeking his morning snuggles. His giggles will be the perfect start to your day, and his hugs will fill your heart with a warmth you never knew was possible. In those moments, your heart will be so full that it feels like life couldn't get any better.

Ally, it might seem unimaginable now, but you are going to fall in love with running. It won't just be a way to keep fit; it'll become your happy place, your therapy, and a huge source of joy. You'll even become a running coach! You'll help other women find their strength and potential through running, and you'll be inspired by their courage and transformations. It will be so rewarding to see how you touch their lives, just as much as they'll touch yours.

In life, you have always been told you're too much, too attention seeking, too loud, too self-absorbed, too caring and compassionate. And yet I know you've lived your whole life thinking you're not enough. Let me tell you, you may love being in the spotlight, because one day you will have to be that shining beacon to attract the amazing and supportive community of women that you run today. You will have to be loud so you can cheer on the women who need to hear you over their own insecurities. What others thought was too much is just enough for the woman that you will become.

Life can be pretty confusing and painful at times, but every little piece of it plays a role in the beautiful story that's unfolding. Just hang in there, okay? Trust that there's a wonderful future waiting for you, filled with love, laughter, and purpose.

Keep going, Ally. You're so much stronger than you realize, and believe me, your best days are still ahead.

With a big hug and lots of love,

Ally, Age 29

It was incredibly therapeutic to write this as I sipped on my morning coffee. Donny and Kylo were in the other room, playing video games, and Summer was sleeping beside me. I really am so grateful to still be alive. I just wish I could tell younger Ally that. I have so many different pieces of advice that I would give her if I could, but more than anything I would just urge her to keep moving forward.

"Even in death, may you be triumphant." -Darren Shan

(featured in the Cirque Du Freak book series)

That may sound like a morbid quote but let me explain the significance. Sometime *AA (after attempt),* I tried to reconnect more with my little sister. We never really spent much time with each other or got along while we were growing up. Zoe was often sick and in and out of the hospital all the time. The majority of that time I spent with my brothers. My sister and I both shared a love for books, and I introduced her to a series that I really loved as a tween, *Cirque Du Freak* by Darren Shan. The series is about a group of vampires who share a belief that to give up, to die on your back, is not only weak, but also disgraceful and shameful. They believed no vampire should go down without a fight. Pride comes from dying on your feet, fighting to the very end. The quote, *"Even in death, may you be triumphant"* encapsulated this belief, and is a prevalent motto among the vampires.

My sister and I took turns reading the books aloud to each other, establishing a closeness that we'd lacked previously. When we came to this line, we both connected to it as it related to our individual lives. For me, it was a reminder of my suicide attempt and the resolve to keep fighting through the darkness. For Zoe, it was a reflection of her ongoing battle with her health issues. We came to an unspoken agreement that we would fight, we would live our lives to the fullest, never giving up or giving in, no matter what that might look like. Years later, we decided to get matching tattoos of these few words, as a constant reminder.

We're both adults now, and it can be easy to let relationships fade when we get busy with our own lives and commitments. This is especially true because we live in different parts of the country and have very different lifestyles. However, over the years, we've made a point to prioritize our connection and sisterly bond. We both understand that maintaining a relationship requires a conscious effort from both parties and in life, we get to choose the loved ones that we keep close. Thus, we hold our weekly Thursday phone date as sacred.

"Level up."

One thing I find fascinating about my relationship with Donny is how we are complete polar opposites. Donny would like to spend the day playing video games, riding motorcycles, or driving remote-controlled cars and then ending the day with some pizza. In contrast, my ideal day involves a long run, curling up with a good book, and ending the afternoon with a peaceful walk on the beach while maintaining a diet with lots of fruit and vegetables. I guess what they say is true. Opposites attract.

Though we are both very different people, with different interests, hobbies, and lifestyles, we have always made time for each other. Going out of our way to support each other. Donny comes to as many of my races as he can, being the best cheerleader, I could ever ask for. In return, I will play video games with him, even though I'm not very good at them. It's great bonding time and allows us to do something interactive together other than watching TV or staring at our phones. Part of my wedding vow actually included that I would always be his Player 2, and we would always help each other level up in life.

Helping each other succeed has always been a defining part of our relationship. When I made the decision to start my business, Donny took on all the financial responsibility for our family while I built up my client base. His support allowed me to pursue my dream. I was then able to reciprocate the enthusiastic support for him when he opened his own motorcycle shop. Rather than working long hours for another company, he now designs and builds custom bikes for the motorcycle speed junkies of South Florida.

Like I said in my letter to my younger self, I wouldn't normally advise anyone to settle down so young in life. I can truly attest that your 20s are for trials and errors and self-discovery. However, there is something undeniably beautiful about having a partner to navigate that exploration with. Knowing there's someone to celebrate successes with and to catch you during stumbles makes the journey that much more fulfilling. There just needs to be a true partnership that allows both people the space to blossom into their own person while still growing together. That's exactly what Donny and I have done over the years. *We have come a long way since the days of ramen noodles and drunken nights.*

As I've become more mindful of my health and fitness journey, one major change in my life has been giving up alcohol. It's been three years since I last had a drink. When I share this with people, I typically get one of two responses. Some people say, *"Wow, congratulations!"* while most others ask, *"Why? What happened?"* Like sobriety had to come from some tragic event. The truth is much simpler: I never liked alcohol in the first place.

When I was a teenager, I drank because I thought it was cool and would help me fit in. I never enjoyed it though. The taste was always unpleasant, and I had to choke it down. I would mix it with sugary sodas or juices to mask the taste, hoping I could drink it without grimacing with every sip. Alcohol did seem to dull the razor-sharp edges of my anxiety and depression though, providing a fleeting escape from reality. There was also a time when I convinced myself that alcohol made me more fun and sociable. I thought it helped me loosen up and made me more likable. But I always hated the way it made me feel.

When I was training for the Ultra Spartan race, the 50-miler, and the World Championships, I was determined to improve my performance. Suddenly, every choice I made was weighed against how it would impact my training. When I was offered a drink, my immediate thought was how it would affect my run the next day. Declining alcohol became an easy choice. *No thanks.* Even with a quick explanation, this decision often surprised and even confused others. I'd get reactions like, *"Oh, are you pregnant?"* or *"One drink won't ruin your run tomorrow!"* It always baffled me because if I turned down a cigarette, no one would think twice. Turning down alcohol continues to be a social crime.

I didn't stop drinking because I had an issue with alcohol itself; I just didn't see any benefit to drinking when I was training so diligently. Alcohol didn't align with my goals, and I didn't want anything to compromise my progress. Then, I actually did get pregnant, followed by breastfeeding. Before I knew it, two years had passed, then three. During that time, I realized that alcohol no longer had a place or purpose in my life. I didn't need to drink just because it can be considered a social norm.

One of the beautiful things about life is that we have the power to make different choices as our lives evolve. Maybe one day, I'll choose to have a drink again. For now, living alcohol-free suits me perfectly, and I'm happy with my decision.

Your Story Matters

Watching *Moving America's Soul on Suicide* at a private viewing, with my husband's arms tightly wrapped around me, was an unbelievably healing experience. As we watched my segment of the film, I felt like I was traveling back through time, reliving all of the dark corners of my past where I'd endured so much shame and regret. But as I watched the documentary and revisited those monumental situations, I was there as a witness to my own strength and resilience. As David Covington reminded me before the viewing, *I've always had that tenacious fire inside of me.* I approached my suicide attempt with the same fearlessness that I do everything else in my life. I found myself there in the packed theater, quietly forgiving my younger self for all of the abuse I put my mind and body through. Each mistake, every helpless and hurting moment, has been a lesson. My history created the mother, the wife, the daughter, the friend, the business owner, the coach, the woman, I am today. Watching my own story on the big screen was a confirmation that every hardship I've faced had a bigger purpose.

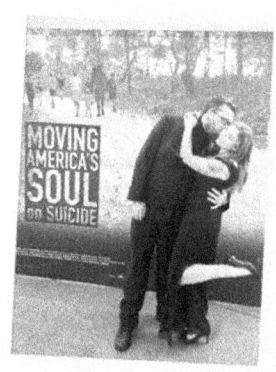

Date night at the film premiere

While this experience was life-changing for me, I hadn't anticipated how deeply my story would resonate with others. I was humbled by the outpouring of emotions from viewers—other young women grappling with suicidal thoughts, mothers who had lost children to suicide, and countless other individuals who saw pieces of their own struggles reflected in my journey. They reached out to say that my story gave them hope, that it made them feel less alone. Or after years of struggling with depression, they were inspired to start running. I hadn't realized just how many people were silently suffering, or that by facing and sharing my own story, I would be able to help in a huge way. My story as a whole is not just a cautionary tale- it shows that there is life on the other side.

When I survived my suicide attempt, the only example I knew of someone else who'd survived an attempt on their own life was Kevin Hines—the young man who miraculously survived after jumping off the Golden Gate Bridge in 2000. His tale is undeniably powerful. Having decided that he could not continue living, he jumped off the famous bridge, but discovered that he still wanted to live only moments after he jumped. But as a teenager, I couldn't relate to his sudden revelation that life was worth living. I didn't wake up from my medically induced coma with a newfound appreciation for life. Instead, I woke up feeling the same despair, the same self-hatred, the same hopelessness that had occupied my mind before my attempt. Surviving a suicide attempt is not the same as living; it's merely the opportunity to begin a complex journey. It would have been helpful to me to have a film with so many storytellers from all walks of life spread the HOPE that there is life worth living after a suicide attempt. *Maybe I wouldn't have even tried to kill myself at all.*

For years I had been afraid to share my story. But now, I hope that as I continue to tell my story, it will reach the ears of the people who need it most. To open doors to deeper and more meaningful conversations regarding mental health and suicide prevention.

One woman I've met in particular comes to mind. Abby started running after leaving an abusive marriage. She found me online through my Facebook group, and she'd been silently watching my posts for months. It wasn't until she saw the link I shared for the film that she sent me a DM asking if we could talk. Abby let me know upfront that she didn't want to waste my time because she wasn't looking for a running coach, but she needed to talk to someone, and she felt a connection because I had shared my story.

Our call lasted longer than either of us expected, and she went on to confide in me that she'd been trapped in an abusive marriage, afraid to leave because she had been completely financially dependent on her husband for most of her adult life. At that point, she questioned if she would ever be able to provide a stable home life for herself and her young son. Abby was at a point where the idea of committing suicide seemed like the best and easiest way out; She only stopped herself because of her child. She knew that she could never leave him alone to deal with his abusive father. Instead of giving up, and giving in, she made the decision to leave. While her husband was at work, she packed up as much as she could carry and took her son to stay at a women's shelter in the next town over. The following months were a struggle. Finding a job, an apartment, and getting back on her feet was made even more difficult by the emotional trauma from years of having to ask her abuser for permission to buy groceries, or even leave the house for any reason.

Abby started running, and that became an outlet for her. Through running, she was able to rebuild her mental, physical, and emotional health. Every time she ran, she was reclaiming her independence, exerting her newfound freedom. She told me that each step she took was a step away from her past and towards a future that she was actively creating for herself. She was redefining her identity. Abby related so much to my story and shared with me that she wished she'd heard my story years before, when she was going through her own darkest moments.

Another person I've connected with as a result of sharing my story in the film was a woman named… well let's call her, Patricia, a 50-something mom whose 18-year-old daughter committed suicide after a lengthy battle with depression and substance abuse. Patricia sent me an email sharing her own story. Her daughter, Lily, had been an active young girl, involved in gymnastics and cheerleading, but had started struggling with peer pressure, bullying, and body dysmorphia when she was only 12 or 13 years old. Patricia had done everything she thought she could, getting Lily into counseling, and paying close attention to how she was spending her free time. Sadly, Lily found friendships with a crowd of older kids who introduced her to drugs and alcohol as a way of dealing with her emotions.

After Lily passed away, Patricia was cleaning her room and found a note on her bedside table, tucked between books. The note simply read, *I love you, Mom.* Patricia told me that she'd struggled with seeing that note and questioning how her daughter could have loved her if she had taken her own life. *Didn't Lily consider how much pain she would cause?* For many years Patricia contemplated joining her daughter on the other side. However, a little voice in the back of her head kept telling her that's not what Lily would have wanted. Only after Patricia heard my story in the film did she realize that her daughter could love her and still feel as though the only option was to take her own life. Patricia finally understood it was never about whether or not Lily loved her mom. Patricia was able to find solace in the fact that Lily was at peace and no longer struggling with her demons. Patricia allowed me to tell her story under an alias in hopes that her story can help other parents and family members cope with the loss of a loved one who has fallen victim to suicide.

As a mom myself, I couldn't imagine being in a relationship where I felt trapped or afraid of my partner, let alone losing one of my children. I know that there's no way I can ever fully understand the pain that these two women have experienced, but I'm so glad that they've found a way to continue on. I'm sure these stories are beyond difficult to share, to hear, and to talk about. Maybe because conversations surrounding mental health and suicide are so difficult, they are even more important to have. The more open we can be with one another, the bigger the ripple of change we can create. The more lives can be saved.

When people ask me for motivational book recommendations, I make it a point to remind them how inspirational their own story is. Sure, there are some amazing books out there filled with incredible tales of men and women overcoming tremendous adversities and accomplishing big audacious goals. These stories can offer a glimmer of inspiration, motivation and even hope when we find ourselves trapped in our own shadows. But in my experience, nothing is as powerful as your own story.

Think about everything you've been through—the struggles, the setbacks, the obstacles you have overcome. Your story is full of raw, real moments that can be way more impactful on your path forward than any book. Your own green hallway will get you through the hardest moments.

I hope you've never had to feel the darkness I've felt. I hope you've never had thoughts of suicide or been in abusive relationships. But if you have, don't forget that's the part of your story that you get to own. You get to tell it in your own way. In the way, I have decided that MY story *is about life.*

Let's keep sharing our stories. We never know who we will inspire or how our experiences might give someone else the courage to keep going. Remember that ripple? It's your turn to drop in a stone, a story.

 # Hope

Suicidal ideation is often misunderstood. It's not always a straightforward wish to die. It can also be a pervasive feeling of being a burden, of believing there's no future worth living for. It can be feeling stuck in a bad situation seeing no hope or possibility for change. There might be the conviction that absolutely no one would care if they were gone. Here's what I've learned: the way to end unbearable pain or feelings of being a burden does not have to result in the ending of a life. We have the power to transform our existence at any moment. Explore the possibility of moving across the country, finding a new passion, starting an interesting hobby, connecting with people outside your social circle, changing careers, starting a business- the possibilities are endless. Even when faced with adversity, we can still choose life.

As an adult, life experiences can show how many ways there are to get out of a difficult situation or allow more resources to make change happen. Teenagers are bound to their parents, school, and maybe even their friend groups. The 1, 2, or even 5 years between now and the freedom of turning 18 can seem like forever. And this feeling of being stuck can make suicide seem like the only available option.

Teen suicide is a crisis that demands our attention. The statistics are staggering and heartbreaking. The World Health Organization, states that suicide is one of the leading causes of death among 15—19-year-olds, according to stats from 2019. Every year more than 5,000 teenagers die from suicide in the United States *(https://www.sccenter.org/programs-and-services/for-teens/teen-suicide-facts/)*. A CDC study analyzing suicidal behaviors and ideation from 2011 to 2021 found that 13% of high school girls had attempted suicide, with 30% having seriously contemplated it. For LGBTQ+ teens, the figures were even higher *(https://www.apa.org/monitor/2023/07/psychologists-preventing-teen-suicide)*.

The reasons behind teen suicide and ideation are complex. Depression, anxiety, bullying, experiencing abuse, parental and personal expectations, feelings of regret, persistent guilt or shame, having low self-esteem, substance abuse, discrimination, the list goes on and on. But at the core of it all is a deep sense of hopelessness and a belief that there is no future worth living for.

Hope, dreams, and goals are the foundations for recovery, regardless of age. They give us something to hold onto, to strive for.

Running became my lifeline. What started as just a goal to run a marathon quickly became my reason to get up in the morning. It opened up an entire world that I became eager to explore. It became the tool that kept me looking to the future, lighting my way through the darkness.

Daring to dream big or going after your goals may be self-help clichés, but it's so easy to get caught up in the mundanity of daily life and let the routine wear us down. We must take time to reflect on our desires and aspirations. I swear this inner work isn't just for Tony Robbins Workshops and self-help.

We don't just stumble upon these life-changing goals and dreams. These ambitions aren't just plastered on billboards waiting for us to notice them. Nope, we've got to roll up our sleeves and dig deep to uncover them, to discover what we enjoy most in life, to explore our true selves and who we want to become.

I once heard a quote that went something like, *"Running a hundred miles in the wrong direction is better than staying still."* At first, I didn't quite get it. I mean, who in their right mind would want to end up stranded after running a hundred miles the wrong way? It sounded like a recipe for disaster! But then it hit me—there's a deeper truth here. When we're moving, even if we're heading in the wrong direction, we're still in motion. We're actively exploring, learning, and discovering what works for us and what doesn't, what we do or don't want in our lives.

Movement, in any form, opens up opportunities. So, go out and run your first race, start nurturing a garden, go back to school, try a new restaurant, live life! Every step, every new adventure, leads us closer to creating our future and inspires and motivates us to achieve new goals, dreams, and ambitions.

To help you figure out your goals, start by asking yourself a few essential questions: What keeps you going? Why do you look forward to waking up tomorrow morning? What truly excites and motivates you? Think about the moments when you felt the most alive and fulfilled. Was it during a particular activity, while achieving a certain milestone, or perhaps when you were helping others?

What comes to mind? Write them down—no filter! Let your imagination run wild.

Once you have a clear vision of what you want to achieve, break these goals down into smaller, more manageable steps. Not only does breaking down a huge goal make it less intimidating and seem more doable, but it gives you a plan. *When I first started running, I wasn't contemplating how to run the entire marathon. I was just focused on mastering my first mile.*

Think of specific actions you can take right now to start moving towards your goals. Maybe it's enrolling in a course, finding a mentor, dedicating time each day to practice a skill, or simply setting aside time for you to continue to explore all that life has to offer.

Life isn't always a smooth ride. There will be bumps and detours, but that's all part of the adventure. Stay focused on your goals, and don't be afraid to tweak your plan if you need to. Surround yourself with cheerleaders—friends, family, or a community of like-minded souls who can keep you motivated.

Don't forget to reflect on your progress. Celebrate your wins, no matter how tiny they might seem. Each milestone is proof of your hard work and dedication. Use those victories as fuel to keep you going and remind yourself why you started this journey.

Ally Robinson

There is No Finish Line

Most people will never understand. They will not understand why runners wake up before the rest of the world has even stirred and subject themselves to hours of grueling training. They see the sweat-soaked shirts and the blistered feet and shake their heads in disbelief. *"You know running is bad for your knees, right?" "The only way you'd get me to run is if a bear was chasing me."*

They may mock us, belittle us, and question our sanity, but they will also never get to experience the transformation and healing that running brings.

For many of us, running is not just a hobby or a form of exercise; it's a way of life—a calling that resonates deep within our souls.

Running isn't for everyone. It's for those who crave the challenge, thrive on the struggle, and refuse to settle for life's modern-day comforts.

And so, we rise before the sun; we embrace the pain and push through the doubt because we know that our reason why—the driving force that keeps us alive, keeps us going—is worth every ounce of effort and sacrifice.

Others might not understand why we lace up our shoes every single day, but I do. I know the allure of the open road, the quiet moments before dawn when the world is still. I embrace the profound sense of accomplishment that comes from pushing through a tough run.

Sleeping in is always an option, so is skipping a workout or choosing an easier path. Quitting will always be an option. Life often tempts us to take the easy way out, to give up when things get tough. But running teaches us that the real victory lies in choosing to keep moving forward, even when every part of us screams to stop. It's about getting out of the zombie haze, taking control of our lives, and making every single step count. We reject the tempting, easy option. Instead, each morning we decide to get up and run, knowing we are choosing our own path and paving a new way. We are choosing to live deliberately, to carve out time for ourselves in the midst of life's chaos, and to move forward with purpose.

After my suicide attempt, I learned that surviving isn't the same as living. It wasn't enough to just exist; I had to actively choose to engage with life every single day, to seek out experiences that brought me joy and fulfillment. Running became a symbol of that choice—a daily commitment to living fully and embracing the journey, no matter how difficult it might be.

I was waiting to *find myself.* I adopted the fake-it-till-you-make-it mentality, thinking that if I just pretended to be fine, eventually I would be. But I never *found* myself. Instead, I chose to create myself. Life is an ever-lasting journey of continuous growth, change, and creation.

One of my favorite films growing up was *Ever After* with Drew Barrymore, a realistic Cinderella story. There's a scene after the ball where the Evil Stepmother and her daughters are anxiously hoping the prince will still choose one of them. Angelica Huston, who plays the Stepmother, says the memorable quote, *"Darling, nothing is final 'til you're dead, and even then, I'm sure God negotiates."* Now when I feel like I am in a tough situation that I'll never get out of, I think about this quote and laugh. Because I know firsthand how quickly life can change in an instant.

One evening after I put the kids to bed, Donny and I watched an interesting documentary about Mount Everest. Donny turned to me and asked, *"Do you want to climb Mount Everest?"*

Having just watched an hour-long program about the bodies of all the ambitious men and women who died on this immense mountain, I wasn't exactly eager to sign up for my potential icy death. The documentary didn't sugarcoat the dangers: frostbite, avalanches, and the likelihood of altitude sickness. None of that seemed like very pleasant ways to die. Then again, Pheidippides, the man who ran to Athens to deliver news of the victory of the battle in Marathon, died shortly after. Creating the legend that eventually started the marathon. Despite this, I still run 26.2 miles... so perhaps death isn't the deterrent for my big goals.

I thought about his question for a moment and responded, *"Do I currently want to spend thousands of dollars battling negative-degree weather and deadly terrain to stand on top of the world? No, not right now. But if you had asked me a few years ago if I wanted to run ultra marathons, I would have said no then, too. So, while my answer is no today, I have no desire to climb Mount Everest... I have no idea what my goals will be tomorrow."*

Running that first marathon felt like scaling my own Everest. At the time, it was such a big goal, each mile was a struggle with my mind and body but crossing that finish line was such an incredible feeling that it made every grueling step worth it. The climb, the struggle, the growth, that's where the magic happens. So, while Mount Everest might not be on my radar today, I embrace the uncertainty and excitement of not knowing where my passions will take me next. And who knows? Maybe one day, standing on top of the world will be just another chapter in my endless race.

I like challenges. I thrive on challenges, especially those that push me to my limits. Running and racing are more than just physical pursuits; they're tests of endurance, resilience, and willpower. I am motivated to find out how fast I can go and how far I can get.

Remember that quote about running 100 miles in the wrong direction? I've taken it to heart, quite literally. In my relentless pursuit to challenge myself, I am currently training for my first 100-mile race. Although the hours of running and training required seem daunting with my already busy schedule and having young children at home who constantly want my attention. I want to see what I'm capable of, both physically and mentally, to test my limits. I want to see what I can really do when the miles stretch on, when my body screams for rest, and when my mind tells me to quit. I know what it feels like to quit. I want to see how far I can push myself without ever quitting again.

Life doesn't get easier; we get stronger. It may be cliche, but it's one that holds undeniable truth. I firmly believe that when I push myself to the limit in running, I'm doing more than just building stamina and endurance, I am preparing myself for life's inevitable challenges. Spartan Races, Ultra Races, and Marathons are situations where I can choose to face suffering, and where I can willingly and *(for the most part*) safely embrace the pain and discomfort of pushing my limitations. It's where I learned to dig deep, to keep going when everything inside me is telling me to stop. And these lessons? They don't stay on the racecourse; they follow me into every aspect of my life.

When life gets tough—and it always does—I know how to handle it because I've been there before. I've faced the doubt, the fear, and the exhaustion, and I've come out the other side, stronger and more resilient. In the end, I want to be physically and mentally strong enough to face all that life has to throw my way.

Every finish line I cross, every medal I earn, is a tangible reminder that I'm still alive, still thriving, and still pushing forward. Whether the race goes as planned or not, I am reminded that the finish line is not the end, but just the beginning of my next big goal. Because in life, unlike in a race, there is no finish line.

In the endless race of life, there is no reason to rush to the end. We can slow down and savor the moments that make life worth living. We can be both driven athletes with ambitious goals and mindful individuals who find joy in the simplicities of life. We can suffer and experience the pleasure of human connection, personal growth, and the endless possibilities that the future holds. We define who we are, make our goals, love fiercely, change the world, and continue finding new reasons to keep running the race of life.

When the idea for this book first came to me, I hesitated. I am only 29 years old, I should wait until I've achieved more, until I'm older, until I cross the finish line of my 100-mile race or have maybe even climbed to the top of Mount Everest, before writing my story. My story isn't even close to being over, how can I write a book if I don't even know how it ends? But I know now that my story will never be over. My story, just like your story, is an ongoing journey, and there is no finish line. Our stories don't need to be wrapped up neatly before they're worth telling. I believe that by sharing my journey now, while I'm still running, still exploring, still growing, I might be able to inspire someone else, someone who needs a little help, a little direction, a little cheering on to start their own race, whatever that looks like for them.

To be continued....

If you or someone you know is experiencing thoughts of suicide or self-harm, please call or text the Suicide and Crisis Lifeline at 988.

To check out the *Moving America's Soul on Suicide* film scan the QR code below.

About the Author

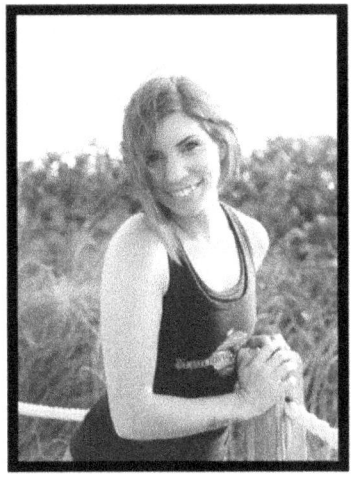

Ally Robinson is a suicide survivor, Spartan Champion, Running Coach, Public Speaker, Podcaster & Author. After surviving her own battles with depression, anxiety, and a nearly fatal suicide attempt at only 15-years-old, Ally realized that while quitting is always an option, it wasn't the one she wanted to choose.

Following her passion for healthy living, Ally obtained her certification as a Personal Trainer, birthed her business, **Something Runderful,** and has been working to coach and empower other unstoppable women since 2019; supporting them through the process of getting faster, stronger, and going further without the overwhelming guesswork that often accompanies the workout game.

Ally's vision extends beyond physical transformation though. She believes that when a woman discovers her strength, when she fiercely and unapologetically goes after her goals, she becomes a beacon of inspiration, influencing not only her immediate circle but also expanding motivation to others around her in a ripple effect that touches hearts and transforms lives.

Robinson currently lives in Miami with her husband, 2 children & a pair of naked cats. She can often be found running at sunrise along the beach, kicking up sand, collecting seashells, and training for her next big race.

For more information about Ally, her podcast, speaking events, or to join **Team Runderful** on a future marathon, visit her website, *www.somethingrunderful.com* via the QR code provided.

If you'd like to share your own story, feel free to contact Ally directly via email at *ally@somethingrunderful.com.*

Ally Robinson

www.ingramcontent.com/pod-product-compliance
Lightning Source LLC
Chambersburg PA
CBHW051629120626
46551CB00014B/2006